Approaches to Semiotics

65

Mouton Publishers
Berlin · New York · Amsterdam

Modes of Medical Instruction

A Semiotic Comparison of Textbooks of Medicine and Popular Home Medical Books

Joan Yess Kahn

Mouton Publishers
Berlin · New York · Amsterdam

Library of Congress Cataloging in Publication Data

Kahn, Joan Yess, 1935-
  Modes of medical instruction.

  (Approaches to semiotics; 65)
  Bibliography: p.
  Includes index.
  1. Medicine–Text-books. 2. Medicine, Popular.
3. Semiotics. I. Title. II. Series.
R118.6.K33 1983 610 83-2379
ISBN 90-279-3070-8

To
Irena Bellert and Irwin Gopnik,
McGill University, Montreal, Quebec

Table of Contents

List of Tables*

*Tables 2 through 19, 29, 40 through 56, and 58, 59 and 60 are accompanied by a companion Graph bearing the same number as the Table, and appearing on the page immediately following it.

Foreword

Basically, *Modes of Medical Instruction* may be properly described as a 'style and contents' comparison involving eight contemporary books of medical instruction—three of which are intended for the instruction of physicians (medical textbooks), and five of which are intended for the instruction of the lay public (popular home medical books). The results of this comparison, however, although interesting in themselves, may also be seen to have significance in the face of reports, widely documented in the various media, concerning the generally frustrating nature of communications exchanged within the context of doctor-patient encounters. In the case of medical students, for example, it is not unreasonable to suppose that they will be inclined to behave, as future physicians, according to the values which are represented in their textbooks. Similarly, lay readers (who are potential patients) are likely to bring to the doctor-patient encounter the values which they receive through the popular media, the latter including popular medical literature. It would seem reasonable, then, that if these two sets of values are discrepant, such a discrepancy may well have consequences with respect to future doctor-patient interactions. The work which follows attempts to make these differences explicit.

Finally, while it may be said that *all* books both reflect as well as perpetuate the social and moral values of the society from which they spring, books of medical instruction, in addition, tend to have profound pragmatic consequences upon the lives of their readers and upon the lives of those who come to be treated by these readers. Clearly, then, the authors, editors and publishers of such books have a responsibility to carefully reflect upon the underlying values upon which such pragmatic instruction is founded.

Preface

The present study, which is a semiotic comparison of textbooks of medicine and popular home medical books, has been organized according to the following assumptions: that the form and contents of such 'books of medical instruction' (a) are most effectively cross-compared by systematically examining certain major structural features which are common to all books, and (b) are most fully interpreted when considered in relation to certain of the social, historical, and critical contexts in which these books occur.

With respect to (a) above, three major 'segments', common to all of the selected books, have been cross-compared: (i) the Text (that portion of a book extending from the beginning of the first chapter until the end of the final chapter), (ii) the Table of Contents, and (iii) the Paratext (everything exclusive of [i] and [ii] above). The reader will note that, following each section which addresses each of the above in Part Two, there appears a corresponding supplement: Supplement A (belonging to that section dealing with the Text), Supplement B (belonging to that section dealing with the Table of Contents), and finally Supplement C (which belongs to that section dealing with the Paratext). Since each of these supplements provides detailed exemplifications or explanations of concepts referred to in their corresponding sections, it was felt that they should be located immediately following each of these sections, rather than at the end of the entire study.

With respect to (b) above, I have undertaken to outline in Part One, Section II, certain social, historical, and critical contexts in which the three selected textbooks of medicine and the five selected popular home medical books occur. One of the principal ways in which the *social* context of these books was determined was through an investigation into the current degree of their dissemination in North America. The results of this investigation appear in Section II: 3. An inquiry into the *historical* context was approached from two aspects: the individual histories or 'genealogies' of each of the selected books, as well as a more general history of books of medical instruction in North America. The results of this inquiry appear in Section II: 4, augmented by material in Appendix A. Next, an inquiry into the *critical* context of the selected books was approached by means of investigating all available critical reviews. Material pertaining to this context appears in Section II: 5, augmented by Appendix B. Finally, in Part One, Section I, which immediately precedes the outline of the argument, I have made an attempt to trace up to the present time the historical development of the term 'semiotics', from its original and exclusively medical application to its subsequent applications, both medical and nonmedical. The tracing of this development was concluded with the following suggestions: (a) that the term 'medical symptomatology' be applied to those 'intraprofessional' works whose main function is the transmission, to members of the medical subculture, of professional skills pertaining to the recognition and interpretation of the signs and symptoms of disease or health; and (b) that the term 'medical semiotics' be reserved for those studies (including the present one) which, in undertaking to analyse various aspects of the medical subculture, bring to that task a systematic application of semiotic theories. With respect to the distinction drawn above, I have thus concluded that section with a 'Selected List of Twentieth Century Works in Medical Symptomatology and Medical Semiotics'.

Immediately following the section described above appears the outline of the argument (Part One, Section I: 2), wherein it is claimed that textbooks may be shown to differ significantly from popular books of medical instruction both in their style and their contents: (a) with respect to style, textbooks may be shown to be formal and authoritative, hence high in accountability, in contrast to popular books, which may be shown to be informal and authoritarian, hence low in accountability (in both cases, style being seen as a function of an assumed relationship between the author and the reader); (b) with respect to contents, it is claimed that textbooks differ from popular books both in terms of their scope (i.e. the types and numbers of topics addressed), as well as in their respective portrayals of *homo medicabilis*, i.e., 'man as the object of a medical description'. The reader will note that statements constituting the arguments outlined in Section II are ultimately addressed individually in Part Three: Conclusions, where the writer has undertaken to substantiate each of them on the basis of evidence drawn from the tables, graphs, supplements and appendices distributed throughout the work.

I wish, at this point, to express special appreciation to three persons who, during the preparation of the Doctoral dissertation upon which the present book is based, have provided me not only with intellectual support, but have been the source of personal encouragement as well. Firstly, I thank my director, Irena Bellert, of the Department of Linguistics and the Graduate Program in Communications,* not only for having suggested the topic of this study to me (for which I am indeed grateful), but for having offered excellent criticism throughout each step of its preparation. Secondly, I wish to thank Irwin Gopnik of the Department of English,* upon whose friendly support and consistently sound critical judgment I have frequently relied ever since he first undertook, several years ago, to direct my Master's thesis. Thirdly, I wish to thank Dr. Hugh Scott, Chief of Medicine, Centre Hospitalier Universitaire, University of Sherbrooke, from whose knowledge and experience in the field of medical education I have benefited greatly.

To Peper Ohlin of the Department of English,* I express thanks for having directed my three doctoral projects, each of which allowed me the opportunity of investigating certain issues which came to be elaborated more fully within the present study. I am also indebted to George Styan of the Department of Mathematics* for his excellent suggestions concerning the presentation of data, to Dr. George Collins of the Montreal Children's Hospital for his many useful comments, and to Dr. Donald Bates of the Department of History of Medicine* for his help in selecting the textbooks appropriate for this study.

In addition, I wish to acknowledge the considerable help I received from several persons in the field of Library Science: Frances Groen and Sandra Emery of the McGill Medical Library, Philip Teigen and Marilyn Fransiszyn of the Osler Library, and Harvey Blackman, graduate student of the School of Library Science, who painstakingly proofread the entire work. I am also grateful to Mildred Solomon for her scrupulous care in typing the manuscript.

Finally, to my husband Amnon, and to our children, Susan and Daniel, I give my special thanks for their support and encouragement.

J.Y.K.
September 1981

*At McGill University, Montreal, Canada.

PART ONE

Books of Medical Instruction

Introduction

1. SEMIOTICS AND MEDICINE: A BRIEF OVERVIEW[1]

Semiotics—the field of theoretic and applied knowledge addressing itself to the study of signs and signifying processes—has been nurtured by three major streams or traditions: a philosophical stream (whose outstanding contributor was the American philosopher, Charles Sanders Peirce, 1839-1914), a linguistic stream (enhanced by the work of Peirce's contemporary, the eminent Swiss linguist, Ferdinand de Saussure, 1857-1913), and, primally, a medical stream (whose ancient source is located in the Hippocratic Corpus, a body of writings which have come to be identified with the Greek physician, Hippocrates, 460-377 B.C.). Thus the relationship between medicine and semiotics can be traced back to Greek antiquity, and Hippocrates has been called not only 'the Father of Greek Medicine', but also 'der Vater und Meister aller Semiotik'.[2]

To properly trace a complete history of medical semiotics requires that one simultaneously undertake a history of symptomatology (a task belonging to the medical historian) and a history of semiotics in general (a task belonging to the historian of the theories of signs). As the writer cannot claim to be either, the following paragraphs are offered only as a general account of how the term 'semiotics', once exclusively applied to a branch of medicine, came to be currently applied to numerous domains of knowledge, of which medicine is but one.

In what was probably its earliest application, the term 'semiotic' (from sēma, 'sign'; sēmeiōtikos, 'observant of signs')[3] referred to that branch of early Greek medicine (of the three branches then established) which dealt with 'the sensible indication of change in the condition of the human body.'[4]

From the writings of the Skeptic philosopher and physician, Sextus Empiricus (ca. A.D. 200-250), information has survived concerning three other early Greek 'physician-semioticians'—the Alexandrian physiologist Erasistratus (310-250 B.C.) and anatomist Herophilus (335-280 B.C.), and the Epicurian, Asclepiades by Bithynia (b. 124 B.C.)—all of whom developed more fully a theory of medical symptomatology.[5]

Galen (ca. A.D. 130-200) identified semiotics as one of six principal branches of medicine, and

'taught that semiotics . . . is to be divided into three parts, "in praereritum cognitionem, in praesentium inspectionem et fututorum providentiam" . . . meaning that its threefold preoccupation must be with diagnostics, focusing on the here and now, and its twin temporal projections into the anamnestic past (i.e. case history) and the prognostic future'.[6]

Under the Epicurians and the Stoics, the theory of signs slowly expanded beyond an exclusive preoccupation with symptoms of disease to include, as well, interpretations of bodily motions as signs of the soul. Thus, for example, not only was fever interpreted as a sign of disease, but blushing was interpreted as a sign of shame, and so on. Also, as is well documented,[7] the Stoics developed sophisticated theories of signs which they applied to logic and language. Hence, the theory of signs gradually evolved 'as a way of proceeding by inference from what is immediately given to the unperceived, and was thus analogous to a doctrine of evidence, particularly [although not exclusively] medical'.[8]

The Greek word, 'semeiotike' was subsequently recruited for use in English philosophical discourse by John Locke (1632-1704), a physician as well as a philosopher. Locke, however, applied the term to logic, which, according to his formulation, constituted one of the three major divisions of all sciences, the other two being 'physica' (i.e. natural philosophy or physics) and 'practica' (i.e. ethics).[9] Locke declared the 'doctrine of signs' to be that branch of the sciences, 'the business whereof is to consider the nature of signs, the mind makes use of for the understanding of things, or conveying its knowledge to others'.[10]

Nearly two centuries later, the English word 'semiotic' appeared in the writings of Charles Sanders Peirce who, perhaps more than any other figure, established semiotics as a discipline. According to Sebeok, Peirce 'undoubtedly took the term "semiotic (semeiotike)" over, with its attendant definition as the " . . . formal doctrine of signs" directly from the usage of Locke'.[11] For Peirce, semiotic(s)[12] constituted a frame of reference for all other studies: 'It has never been in my power to study anything—mathematics, ethics, metaphysics, gravitation, thermodynamics, optics, chemistry, comparative anatomy, astronomy, pyschology, phonetics, economic, history of science, whist, men and women, wine, metrology—except as a study of semiotic . . .'.[13]

In his writings, Peirce emphasized the triadic nature of the signifying process.[14] With respect to medicine, two of his theoretic formulations hold particular interest: (1) his classification of varieties of signs based upon the nature of the relationship between an object and its sign, thus: 'icons' (the relationship between object and sign being that of resemblance of qualities), 'symbols' (the relationship between object and sign being arbitrated purely through a conventional law), and 'indexes' or 'indices' (the relationship between object and sign being that of contiguity, for example, the weather-vane indicating the direction of the wind, the lowering of a column of mercury in a barometer, and a symptom[15] of illness); (2) his distinction between 'token' and 'type' which, while initially applied to words,[16] may, in the opinion of the writer, be applied as well to 'symptom-tokens' (such as an actual instance of a cough or nausea), and 'symptom-types' (i.e. the classes of such symptoms).

Influenced by Peirce, the American psychologist Charles W. Morris (1901-1979) undertook further work in developing a general theory of signs, and established the now widely-used tripartite division of semiotics into semantics, pragmatics, and syntax[17] (later propagated by Carnap).[18] Morris also applied himself to the task of distinguishing animal sign-behavior from that of man,[19] a distinction which is now expressed in a current division of semiotics into 'anthroposemiotics', which concerns itself with 'the totality of man's species-specific signaling systems'[20] and 'zoosemiotics', 'which encompasses the study of animal communication in the broadest sense.[21] An emerging third domain, which cuts across both anthroposemiotics and zoosemiotics is that of 'endosemiotics' (still in a fledgling state), 'which studies cybernetic systems within the [human or animal] body',[22] particularly with respect to 'the coding and transmission of information inside,'[23] an area of study that is linked in a very obvious way with the field of medicine.

In contrast to the 'Locke-Peirce-Morris' (or 'philosophical-psychological') stream of semiotics, there emerged a third and highly influential linguistic stream, whose progenitor was the Swiss linguist, Ferdinand de Saussure:

Language is a system of signs that express ideas, and is therefore comparable to a system of writing, the alphabet of deaf-mutes, symbolic rites, polite formulas, military signals, etc. But it is the most important of all these systems.

A science that studies the life of signs within society is conceivable; . . . I shall call it *semiology* (from Greek sēmeîon 'sign'). Semiology would show what constitutes signs, what laws govern them . . . . Linguistics is only a part of the general science of semiology; the laws discovered by semiology will be applicable to linguistics, and the latter will circumscribe a well-defined area within the mass of anthropological facts.[24]

Although Saussure acknowledges a broad social application of his science of semiology, his efforts were directed mainly toward language. Thus, certain of his theoretic contributions have relevance for medicine[25] largely through their application to what may be called 'medical English' (for example, his distinctions between 'langue' and 'parole', between 'synchrony' and 'diachrony', between 'syntagmatics' and 'paradigmatics', as well as his emphasis upon the double aspect of the sign, namely, 'signifier' and 'signified').

According to Sebeok, '[a] rapprochement between the general theory of signs and the medical praxis involving signs is rather recent, in no small part stimulated by the distinguished work of Michel Foucault'.[26] Besides Foucault, Sebeok cites other post-Saussurean 'structuralists', such as the literary critic, Rolland Barthes, and the psychiatrist and psychoanalyst, Jacques Lacan, as having demonstrated a special interest in the interface between medicine and semiotics. Sebeok cites as well the North American contributions made by two psychiatrists, Jurgen Ruesch and Harley Shands, and the work of the Swiss-born philosopher, Eugen Bar, all of whose works are heavily informed by an interest both in theories of 'disturbed communication', as well as in the clinical manifestations (both verbal and psychosomatic) of such disturbances.

Another contemporary North American 'descendant' of the linguistics stream is Naomi Sager, who has authored and coauthored numerous works in the field of medical linguistics, particularly with respect to computerized studies of patients' medical records.

In concluding this section, the following suggestion is proposed for the reader's consideration:

Concerning all persons in the medical and health professions[27] directly or indirectly engaged in the recognition of signs and symptoms of physical and psychological 'health' and 'disease' in actual individuals, it is suggested that such written (or graphic) contributions which they make strictly with respect to the above, be said to belong to the general domain of *medical symptomatology*:[28] Such works, characteristically, would be designed for the communication of professional knowledge and skills to the author's coprofessionals, and to the next generation of those electing to work in the medical (or paramedical) subculture.

Works in *medical semiotics,* on the other hand (authored either by professionals or nonprofessionals), might then include any of the following: the semiotics of doctor-patient encounters in clinics, in doctors' offices, or in other contexts (e.g. insurance examinations, army entrance examinations, etc.), the semiotics of hospital design in relation to staff-patient interactions, the semiotics of operating room rituals,[29] the semiotics of medical iconography in painting, the semiotics of media productions (radio, cinema, or television) dealing with medical subject matter, the semiotics of drug advertising addressed to doctors,[30] the semiotics of patients' medical records,[31] the semiotics of psychoanalytic discourse,[32] the semiotics of books of medical instruction (the topic of the present study), and all other such cultural studies in which semiotic theories are applied to the domain of medicine.

In the opinion of the writer, a general acknowledgement of a clear distinction between works in medical symptomatology and works in medical semiotics would help foster a 'healthy' dialogue between those who, because of their training, are likely to express the value system of the medical subculture, and those who, by virtue of being outside that subculture, can speak from alternative perspectives. With respect to the distinction drawn above, the reader will find below a selected list of works.

SELECTED LIST[33] OF TWENTIETH CENTURY WORKS IN MEDICAL SYMPTOMATOLOGY AND MEDICAL SEMIOTICS

A. Medical symptomatology

Hamilton Bailey, *Demonstrations of Physical Signs in Clinical Surgery* (Bristol: Wright, 1967).

Julius Bauer, *Differential Diagnosis of Internal Diseases, Clinical Analysis and Syntheses of Symptoms and Signs on Pathophysiological Basis*, 3rd rev. and enl. ed. (New York: Grune, 1967).

D.R. Collins, *Illustrated Diagnosis of Systemic Diseases* (Philadelphia: Lippincott, 1972).
Illustrated Diagnosis of Localized Diseases (Philadelphia: Lippincott, 1974).

F.G. Crookshank, *Individual Diagnosis* (London: Routledge and Kegan Paul, 1930).

Alan Edward David and T.D. Bolin, *Symptom Analysis and Physical Diagnosis* (Rushcutters Bay, Australia: Pergamon, 1977).

Alvin Feinstein, *Clinical Judgment* (Baltimore: Williams and Wilkins, 1967).

R.R. Grinker and A. Robbins, *Psychosomatic Casebook* (New York: Blackiston, 1954).

Francis Dudley Hart, ed., *French's Index of Differential Diagnosis*, 10th ed. (Baltimore: Williams and Wilkins, 1973).

Abner McGehee Harvey and J. Bordley, *Differential Diagnosis: The Interpretation of Clinical Evidence*, 2nd ed. (Philadelphia: Saunders, 1970).

Jacques Lacan, *The Language of Self: The Function of Language in Psychoanalysis*, trans. with notes and commentary by A. Wilden (Baltimore: Johns Hopkins University Press, 1958).

Patrick Mahoney, 'Towards a formalist approach to dreams', *International Review of Psychoanalysis* 4 (1977): 83-98.

—'The place of psychoanalytic treatment in the history of discourse', *Psychoanalysis and Contemporary Thought* 2 (1979): 77-111.

—'The boundaries of free association', *Psychoanalysis and Contemporary Thought* 2 (1979).

—'Towards the understanding of translation in pyschoanalysis', *Journal of the American Psychoanalytic Association* 28 (1980).

Patrick Mahoney and Rajendra Singh, 'The interpretation of dreams, semiology and Chomskian linguistics: A radical critique', *Psychoanalytic Study of the Child* 30 (1975): 221-241.

Patrick Mahoney and Rajendra Singh, 'Critical review of Edison's *Language and Interpretation*', in *Psychoanalysis and Contemporary Thought* (1980).

Peter Mills, *The Significance of Physical Signs in Medicine* (London: H.K. Lewis, 1971).

John A. Prior and Jack S. Silberstein, *Physical Diagnosis: The History and Examination of the Patient*, 4th ed. (St. Louis: Mosby, 1973).

Jurgen Ruesch, *Disturbed Communication: The Clinical Assessment of Normal and Pathological Communicative Behaviour* (New York: Norton, 1957).

—*Therapeutic Communication* (New York: Norton, 1961).

Jurgen Ruesch and Gregory Bateson, *Communication: The Social Matrix of Psychiatry* (New York: Norton, 1951).

M. Thorek, *The Face in Health and Disease* (Philadelphia: Davis, 1946).

University of Edinburgh, Faculty of Medicine, *Clinical Examination: A Textbook for Students and Doctors by Teachers of the Edinburgh Medical School*, ed. John MacLeod, 4th ed. (Edinburgh: Churchill Livingstone, 1976).

B. *Medical semiotics*

Eugen Bar, 'The language of the unconscious according to Jacques Lacan', *Semiotica* 3 (1971): 241-268.

—*Semiotic Approaches to Psychotherapy*. Studies in Semiotics 1 (Bloomington: Research Center for Language and Semiotic Studies, 1975).

Roland Barthes, 'Semiologie et medicine', in *Les sciences de la folie*, ed. Roger Bastide (Paris: Mouton, 1972), pp. 37-46.

Lucille Hollander Blum, *Reading Between the Lines: Doctor-Patient Communication* (New York: International Universities Press, 1972).

Eugen Celan and Solomon Marcus, " Le diagnostic comme langage', *Cahiers de Linguistique* 10 (1973).

F.G. Crookshank, 'The importance of a theory of signs and a critique of language in the study of medicine', in C.K. Ogden and I.A. Richards, *The Meaning of Meaning* (New York: Harcourt, Brace and World, 1923).

Horacio Fabrega, Jr., 'Medical anthropology', in *Biennial Review of Anthropology*, ed. Bernard J. Siegel (Stanford, Calif.: Stanford University Press, 1971).

Michel Foucault, *The Birth of the Clinic: An Archaeology of Medical Perception*, trans. by A.M. Sheridan Smith (New York: Random House, 1975).

R. Grishman and L. Hirschman, 'Question answering from natural language medical data bases', *Artificial Intelligence II* (1978): 25-43.

L. Hirschman and R. Grishman, 'Fact retrieval from natural language medical records', *IFIP World Conference Series on Medical Informatics 2*, eds. D.B. Shires and H. Wolf (Amsterdam, 1977), pp. 247-251.

L. Hirschman, R. Grishman, and N. Sager, 'From text to structured information: Automatic processing of medical reports', *AFIPS Conference Proceedings 45* (Montvale, New Jersey: AFIPS Press, 1976): 267-275. (National Computer Conference, 1976.)

L. Hirschman, N. Sager and M. Lyman, 'Automatic application health care criteria to narrative patient records', *Proceedings of the Third Annual Symposium on Computer Application in Medical Care* (in press).

Joan Y. Kahn, 'A diagnostic semiotic', *Semiotica* 22 (1978): 75-104.

Kathleen Lewis, 'Conference on language and medicine', *Language Sciences* 12 (1970): 14-16.

Peter F. Ostwald, 'Discussion session on psychiatry', in *Approaches to Semiotics: Cultural Anthropology, Education, Linguistics, Psychiatry, Psychology*, eds. Thomas A. Sebeok, Alfred S. Hayes, and Mary Catherine Bateson (The Hague: Mouton, 1964).

___'How the patient communicates about disease with the doctor', in *Approaches to Semiotics: Cultural Anthropology, Education, Linguistics, Psychiatry, Psychology*, eds. Thomas A. Sebeok, Alfred S. Hayes, and Mary Catherine Bateson (The Hague: Mouton, 1964), pp. 11-34, with discussion, pp. 35-49.

___'Symptoms, diagnosis and concepts of disease: Some comments on the semiotics of patient-physician communication', *Social Science Information* 7 (1968): 95-106.

Jurgen Ruesch, *Semiotic Approaches to Human Relations*. Approaches to Semiotics 25 (The Hague: Mouton, 1972).

N. Sager, 'Natural language information formatting: The automatic conversion of texts to a structured data base', in *Advances in Computers 17*, ed. M.C. Yovits (New York: Academic Press, 1978), pp. 89-162.

N. Sager and M. Lyman, "Computerized language processing: implications for health care evaluation', *Medical Record News* 49 (June 1978): 20-30.

N. Sager, L. Hirschman, R. Grishman, and C. Insolio, 'Transforming medical records into a structured data base', in D. Waltz, *Natural Language Interfaces, ACM-SIGART Newsletter* no. 61 (February 1977): 38-39.

N. Sager, L. Hirschman, and M. Lyman, 'Computerized language processing for multiple use of narrative discharge summaries', in *Proceedings of the Second Annual Symposium on Computer Applications in Medical Care,* ed. F.H. Orthner (New York: IEEE, 1978), pp. 330-343.

Harley C. Shands, 'Momentary deity and personal myth: A semiotic inquiry using recorded psychotherapeutic material', *Semiotica* 2 (1970): 1-34.

__Semiotic Approaches to Psychiatry.* Approaches to Semiotics 2 (The Hague: Mouton, 1970).

__The War with Words: Structure and Transcendence.* Approaches to Semiotics 12 (The Hague: Mouton, 1971).

Harley C. Shands and James D. Meltzer, 'Clinical semiotics', *Language Sciences* 38 (1975): 21-24.

Kathryn Vance Staiano, 'A semiotic definition of illness', paper presented at the Third Annual Meeting of the Semiotic Society of America, Providence, Rhode Island, Fall, 1978.

Lawrence L. Weed, *Medical Records, Medical Education and Patient Care: The Problem-Oriented Record as a Basic Tool* (Cleveland: The Press of Western Reserve University, 1969).

2.   OUTLINE OF ARGUMENT: HOMO MEDICABILIS DEFINED

The myths of Hygeia and Asclepius symbolize the never-ending oscillation between two different points of view in medicine. For the worshippers of Hygeia, health is the natural order of things, a positive attribute to which men are entitled if they govern their lives wisely. According to them, the most important function of medicine is to discover and teach the natural laws which will ensure to man a healthy mind in a healthy body. More skeptical or wiser in the ways of the world, the followers of Asclepiades believe that the chief role of the physician is to treat disease, to restore health by correcting any imperfection caused by the accidents of birth or of life. . . . In one form or another these two complementary aspects of medicine have always existed simultaneously in all civilizations. . .[34]

A systematic cross-comparison has been undertaken between three contemporary North American textbooks of medicine and five popular home medical books, especially in terms of their constituent signs, but also in terms of certain social, historical, and critical contexts in which these books may be located.

By citing evidence drawn from this comparison, I shall attempt to demonstrate how the two groups of 'books of medical instruction' indicated above may be clearly differentiated on the levels of form and contents.

With respect to form, I shall attempt to show that textbooks, as a group, are formal, authoritative, and high in accountability, in contrast to popular books which, as a group, are informal, authoritarian, and low in accountability. In each case, the form is interpreted as a function of an assumed relationship between the writer and the reader: in the case of textbooks, that of 'master' to 'apprentice', and in the case of popular books, that of 'friendly consultant' to 'concerned client'.

Concerning contents, I will try to show that textbooks and popular books differ not only in terms of their scope (i.e. in terms of the kinds and numbers of topics which are addressed), but also in terms of the way in which each group tends to portray *homo medicabilis,* or, man as the object of a medical description.

The scope of these books has been investigated from a broad as well as a narrow perspective: broadly, in terms of the scope of an entire book (as indicated by the set of main headings in its Table of Contents), and narrowly, in terms of the scope of a particular part of a book, i.e. a Disease Description (as indicated by the set of bold-type headings interspersed throughout such a description). In the case of this study, descriptions selected for cross-comparison are of the disease, diabetes mellitus.

Homo medicabilis, i.e. man as the object of a medical description, may be best understood as: man as described with respect to his role as a potential or actual 'bearer' of the signs of health or disease, or, as a potential or actual participant in diagnostic and therapeutic processes. Since no coherent description of *homo medicabilis* appears in any of the books, it was necessary to construct one on the basis of a number of characteristics observed in all eight selected books, in much the same way as a psychologist, for example, in attempting to describe various clusters of characteristics observed in a population of human subjects, constructs a 'profile' of a certain 'personality-type'. However, it is important to emphasize that, in the same way that not every human subject whom the psychologist so typifies necessarily possesses every feature of the 'type', so also is it the case that not every textbook displays all features of *homo medicabilis* Type T,[35] and that not every popular book displays all features of *homo medicabilis* Type P.[36]

I shall try to show, however, that, as a group, textbooks tend to describe *homo medicabilis* as a biological system with constituent subsystems, each in turn comprised of organic and suborganic components, the functions or malfunctions of which are accounted for largely in terms of measurable alterations of biochemical values; moreover, that these books generally assume that not only is this system highly predisposed toward such aberrant states as diseases and disorders, but that the appropriate method of diagnosing and correcting such states involves carefully measured biochemical agents, the administration and use of which are to be carried out under the close external supervision and control of a licensed medical doctor.

I shall further attempt to demonstrate that popular books, in contrast, tend to portray *homo medicabilis* as a body endowed with a mind; a body, moreover, which is described largely in terms of its internal and external 'parts'; secondly, that *homo medicabilis* Type P is less often described as a 'patient' than as a 'person', one who is clearly located within the context of a family and social life; finally, that not only is his given state assumed to be that of health rather than disease, but that both the prevention of disease, as well as the relief of many of its symptoms, are assumed to be highly amenable to his own self-regulation, especially through such 'natural' means as diet, dietary supplements, massage, rest, and exercise.

Thus it will be argued that since the selected popular books (notwithstanding their clear acknowledgment of the existence of specific diseases) emphasize both the given fact of health as well as the efficacy of prevention, they are more optimistic in their outlook than are the selected textbooks. Furthermore, to the degree that they encourage their readers to take a greater role in 'governing' their own biological states, *homo medicabilis* Type P is assigned a greater degree of autonomy than is his textbook counterpart.

I shall try to substantiate these arguments from a variety of data selected from three segments of the books: the Table of Contents, the Text (all material extending from the beginning of the first to the end of the final chapter), and the Paratext (everything else). These three divisions have been used as an organizing principle in the presentation of data in Part Two.

However, my conclusions in Part Three will have been founded not only upon data drawn from the three segments indicated above, but, as well, upon data drawn from various sources outside the selected books, such as book reviews, biographical data pertaining to the authors or editors, historical data pertaining to the 'genealogy' of each book, and so on.

This 'broad spectrum' approach to an understanding of the significant differences in the form and the contents of textbooks of medicine as compared to popular home medical books assumes the following:

1. that the question of form may be treated not only as the form of an entire book (as distinct from a more conventional treatment of form which is restricted to the Text as defined above), but also, as the characteristic form of an identified genre, namely, books of medical instruction, of which two sub-types may be clearly distinguished.

2. that the concept of *homo medicabilis,* insofar as its conception is the outcome of an investigation not only of the eight selected books, but also, of a variety of medical writings from other sources, may be usefully applied as a focal concept, both in the case of the present study, as well as (it is suggested) in the case of subsequent historical comparisons (e.g. a comparison of sixteenth century and twentieth century *homo medicabilis*), or of subsequent cross-cultural studies (e.g. a comparison of *homo medicabilis 'africanus'* and *homo medicabilis 'americanus'*).

3. that this writer's approach to books of medical instruction is that they constitute highly complex sign-systems which, when investigated by the medical semiotician, are most fully interpreted in relation to the cultural and ideological contexts from which they arise.

Thus, for the reasons just stated, although the main body of this study investigates the selected books with respect to their constituent signs (Part Two), and for the purpose of concluding differences in form and contents (Part Three), an attempt has been made to indicate, albeit briefly (Part One), at least some of the social, historical, and critical contexts in which the selected books occur.

NOTES

1. This section has been largely informed by material found in Thomas A. Sebeok, *Studies in Semiotics: Contributions to the Doctrine of Signs* (Bloomington: Indiana University Press, 1976), especially Chapter 1, 'Semiotics: A survey of the state of the art', Chapter 2, ' "Semiotics" and its congeners', Chapter 8, 'Six species of signs: Some propositions and strictures', and Chapter 10, 'The semiotic web: A chronicle of prejudices'.

2. Sebeok 1976: 126 (attributed to Rudolph Kleinpaul, *Sprache ohne Worte: Idee einer allgemeinen Wissenschaft der Sprache* [Leipzig: Friedrich, 1888]. Reprinted in *Approaches to Semiotics* 19 [The Hague: Mouton, 1972]).

3. Sebeok 1976: 48.

4. Sebeok 1976: 3-4. This narrower meaning of 'semiotics' still survives in the word 'symptomatology' (in English-speaking countries) and 'semeiology' or 'semiology' (in certain European countries).

   Such "sensible indications" have long been distinguished on the basis of the role-identity of the individual for whom the 'indications' are 'sensible': when sensible to a patient (or to a prospective patient), i.e. 'subjectively', such indications are generally referred to as 'symptoms'; when sensible to a physician (or to a surrogate-physician, such as a parent or spouse), i.e. 'objectively', such indications are generally referred to as 'signs'. However, the distinction between 'symptom' and 'sign', drawn as above, does not hold universally.

5. Sebeok 1976: 125.

6. Sebeok 1976: 182, citing Claudius Galenus, *Opera Omnia* 14 (Hildesheim: Georg Olms, s.d.).
7. See, for example, Benson Mates, *Stoic Logic* (Berkeley: University of California Press, 1953).
8. Sebeok 1976: 47.
9. John Locke, *An Essay Concerning Human Understanding,* abridged and edited by A.D. Woozley (New York: William Collins and Sons, 1964), p. 442.
10. Locke 1964: 443.
11. Sebeok 1976: 48-49.
12. According to Sebeok, neither Peirce nor his 'successor', Charles W. Morris, used the now current term 'semiotics' in any of their writings.
13. I.C. Lieb, ed., *Charles S. Peirce's Letters to Lady Welby* (New Haven: Whitlock's, 1953), p. 32.
14. According to Peirce, this process involves a sign (or a First), an object (or a Second), and an interpretant (or a Third).
15. Sebeok defines a symptom as 'a compulsive, automatic, nonarbitrary sign, such that the signifier is coupled with the signified in the manner of a natural link'. See Sebeok 1976: 124.
16. 'The total number of words in a text gives us the number of tokens; the total number of different words gives the number of types'. Oswald Ducrot and Tzvetan Todorov, eds., *Encyclopedic Dictionary of the Sciences of Language,* trans. by Catherine Porter (Baltimore and London: The Johns Hopkins University Press, 1979), p. 105.
17. Charles W. Morris, *Foundations of the Theory of Signs,* vol. 1, no. 1 (Chicago: University of Chicago Press, 1970), pp. 6-7.
18. Sebeok 1976: 157.
19. Sebeok 1976: x.
20. Sebeok 1976: 3.
21. Sebeok 1976: 3.
22. Sebeok 1976: 3.
23. Sebeok 1976: 3.
24. Ferdinand de Saussure, *Course in General Linguistics* (New York: McGraw-Hill, 1966), p. 16.
25. The *Course* contains no mention of medical signs or symptoms whatsoever.
26. Sebeok 1976: 126.
27. These persons might be doctors, nurses, psychologists, psychoanalysts, physiotherapists, occupational therapists, speech therapists, sex therapists, family therapists, and so on.
28. Thus, to the degree that any work (either in diagnostics, prognostics, history-taking, prevention, or even therapeutics) takes into account the symptoms and signs of disease (including signs which are apprehended by technological artifacts), such works (at least from the viewpoint of the semiotician) may be said to belong to the field of medical symptomatology. It is of interest to note that the current edition of MeSH (i.e. *Medical Subject Headings*) does not have a heading for 'Symptomatology'.
29. The writer has often been struck by the similarities or behavior towards objects on the part of those who are motivated by the distinction between 'contaminated' and 'sterile' and those who are motivated by the distinction between 'profane' and 'sacred'.

30. Donald Theall, former Chairman of the Graduate Program in Communications at McGill University, has initiated some research in this area.
31. With respect to patients' medical records, see the respective works of Naomi Sager and the writer on the 'Selected List' above.
32. With respect to psychonalytic discourse, see the respective works of Jacques Lacan, Harley Shands, Eugen Bar and Patrick Mahoney in the 'Selected List' above.
33. The writer apologizes for inadvertant omissions of writings by other authors working in the fields of medical symptomatology or medical semiotics. Moreover, she wishes to state that the inclusion of this 'List' is not intended to imply a personal familiarity with every one of the cited works. Finally, with respect to certain works authored by professional psychiatrists, their location under one or the other heading category was based upon either the title of the work or the title of the journal in which the work was published.
34. Rene Dubos, *Mirage of Health* (New York: Doubleday, 1959), pp. 114-115.
35. For Textbook type.
36. For Popular type.

Eight Books of Medical Instruction

1. SELECTION CRITERIA

The criteria used in the selection of the eight books of medical instruction for this investigation were the following:

a. that they be designed with an intention to teach, inform, and instruct[1] the North American reader with respect to some aspects of the broad subject of general medicine (albeit at different levels of complexity, for different ends, and with an anticipation of different kinds of readers);
b. that they be current;[2]
c. that they be published in North America and written in the English language;[3]
d. that they be currently disseminated[4] in North America.

2. CODED LIST OF SELECTED BOOKS

a. *Texbooks of medicine*

T-1[5] - *Harrison's Principles of Internal Medicine,* 8th ed. Ed. by G.W. Thorn. (New York: McGraw-Hill, 1977).
T-2 - *Textbook of Medicine,* 14th ed. Ed. by P.B. Beeson and W. McDermott. (Philadelphia: Saunders, 1975).
T-3 - *The Principles and Practice of Medicine,* 19th ed. Ed. by A.M. Harvey. (New York: Appleton-Century-Crofts, 1976).

b. *Popular home medical books*

P-1 - *Better Homes and Gardens Family Medical Guide,* Rev. ed. Ed. by D.G. Cooley. (New York: Meredith, 1977).

P-2   - *Doctor Homola's Natural Health Remedies.* By Samuel Homola, D.C. (West Nyack, N.Y.: Parker, 1973).

P-3   - *The Family Book of Preventive Medicine: How to Stay Well all the Time.* By Benjamin Miller, M.D. and Laurence Galton. (New York: Simon and Schuster, 1971).

P-4   - *The Encyclopedia of Common Diseases.* By Charles Gerras et al. (Emmaus, Penn.: Rodale, 1976).

P-5   - *The Handy Home Medical Adviser and Concise Medical Encyclopedia,* New rev. ed. Ed. by Morris Fishbein, M.D. (New York: Doubleday, 1973).

3.   DISSEMINATION OF THE SELECTED BOOKS OF MEDICAL INSTRUCTION IN NORTH AMERICA

a.   *Textbooks: A postal survey of medical libraries*

In order to determine the extent of dissemination and use within North American medical school libraries of the three textbooks of medicine under consideration, 136 survey questionnaires were sent out to the reference librarians of those medical libraries associated with North American medical schools, as listed in *Medical School Admission Requirements 1979-1980* (Washington: Association of American Colleges, 1978). Of the 136 questionnaires sent out, 130 responses were obtained, yielding a response rate of 95.6%. The questionnaire was designed as follows:

Part A.   The following textbooks are *available as basic reference material* in our library:
1.   *Harrison's Principles of Internal Medicine, ed. 8,* ed. by G.W. Thorn et al. . . . . . . YES . . . . . NO
2.   *Textbook of Medicine, ed. 14,* ed. by P.B. Beeson and W. McDermott . . . . YES . . . . . NO
3.   *The Principles and Practice of Medicine, ed. 19,* ed. by A. McG. Harvey et al. . . . . . . YES . . . . . NO
Part B.   Of the three, I would *estimate* that (1 2 3) is most frequently consulted, followed by (1 2 3).[6]

Regarding Part A of the questionnaire, which was completed by 130 (100%) of the respondents, the following pattern of textbook dissemination emerged:

Textbook	No. of responding medical school library locations in which textbook is designated as basic reference material
Harrison's Principles of Internal Medicine, 8th edition (CODE = T-1)	130 (100% of the respondents)
Textbook of Medicine, 14th edition (CODE = T-2)	130 (100% of the respondents)
The Principles and Practice of Medicine, 19th edition (CODE = T-3)	120 (92.3% of the respondents)

Regarding Part B of the questionnaire, which was completed by 124 of the 130 respondents (95.4%), the pattern of library use which emerged was as follows:

The most frequently consulted textbook was:
T-1   (according to 111, or 89.5% of the respondents to Part B)
T-2   (according to 11, or 8.9% of the respondents to Part B)
T-3   (according to 1, or 0.8% of the respondents to Part B)
All consulted equally (according to 1, or 0.8% of the respondents to Part B)

The second most frequently consulted textbook was:
T-2   (according to 85, or 68.5% of the respondents to Part B)
T-3   (according to 26, or 21.0% of the respondents to Part B)
T-1   (according to 9, or 7.3% of the respondents to Part B)
Other responses (from 4, or 3.2% of the respondents to Part B)

In all cases in which the respondents claimed to carry only two of the three textbooks as basic reference material (10 out of 130, or 7.7% of the respondents), the selected books were always T-1 and T-2, but never T-3. In these 10 library locations, the pattern of library use was as follows:

Order of frequency of textbook use	No. of '2-book locations' (total = 10)
T-1, T-2	In 9 of 10 locations (90%)
T-2, T-1	In 1 of 10 locations (10%)

In all cases in which the respondents claimed to carry all three textbooks as basic reference material (120 out of 130, or 92.3% of the respondents), the following patterns of library use emerged, based, however, upon only 114 responses (as six of the responses were invalid):

Order of frequency of textbook use	No. of '3-book locations' (total = 114)
T-1, T-2	75 (65.8% of locations)
T-1, T-3	24 (21.1% of locations)
T-2, T-1	8 (7.0% of locations)
T-2, T-3	2 (1.7% of locations)
T-3, T-2	1 (0.9% of locations)
T-3, T-1	0
Other variations	4 (3.5% of locations)

The results of the postal survey of medical libraries clearly indicate that all three textbooks of medicine which have been selected for this investigation enjoy an extraordinarily wide degree of dissemination within North American medical school libraries, with T-1 (Harrison's) and T-2 (Beeson and McDermott) available as basic reference material in at least 95.6% of all such libraries, and in 100% of the responding libraries. T-3 (Harvey's) was almost as widely disseminated as were the other two, available as basic reference material in at least 88.2% of all such libraries, and 92.3% of the responding libraries.

With respect to the frequency with which these three textbooks of medicine were consulted, based upon estimations made by medical reference librarians, T-1 (Harrison's) proved by far to be the most frequently consulted, estimated as such in 90% of the 2-book locations, and in 86% of the 3-book locations. Its closest 'rival', T-2 (Beeson and McDermott) was claimed to be the most frequently consulted in 10% of the 2-book locations, and in 8.8% of the 3-book locations. Finally, T-3 (Harvey's) was absent in every 2-book location, and was claimed to be most frequently consulted in only 0.9% of the 3-book locations.

As to which textbook of medicine was estimated as the second most frequently consulted, T-2 (Beeson and McDermott) was selected in 90% of the 2-book locations, and in 66.6% of the 3-book locations. The closest 'rival' for second place was found to be T-3 which, while absent from all 2-book locations, was designated as the second most frequently consulted textbook of medicine in 22.8% of all 3-book locations. T-1 (Harrison's) occupied second place in only 1% of the 2-book locations, and in 7% of the 3-book locations. Finally, in only one of the 120 3-book locations was it claimed that all three textbooks of medicine were consulted with equal frequency.

There appeared to be no significant correlation between the geographic location of the medical school libraries involved, and the order of frequency of textbook use.

Results of the postal survey addressed to North American medical school librarians make it evident that the three selected textbooks are widely distributed and read, hence are probably highly influential in the current dissemination of knowledge related to internal medicine. Recently, however, a new kind of textbook of medicine has been published: *Scientific American Medicine,* edited by E. Rubenstein and D.D. Federman (New York: Scientific American, 1978). This book, coauthored by 27 physicians from Stanford and Harvard, appears in a two-volume, loose-leaf format which, according to the editors, permits its readers to keep abreast of current developments by means of updated sections and indexes which are sent out monthly by the publishers. In addition, this textbook provides a mechanism whereby the reader may obtain credits in continuing medical education.[7] Whether this format will gain as wide an audience as the traditionally bound textbooks will remain to be seen.

b.   *Popular home medical books: Market research*

Letters were written to the American publishers of the five selected popular home medical books, requesting information pertaining to sales of the selected books in North America. None, however, responded to this request.

Personal communication with eight Canadian booksellers, and five American booksellers indicated that most popular home medical books, of the type that have been selected for this investigation, are (to use their phrase) 'good sellers'.

The only specific figures that this investigator was able to obtain came from the Canadian subsidiary of the American firm that published *The Handy Home Medical Adviser and Concise Medical Encyclopedia* (P-5). A representative of this subsidiary claimed that this book has sold a minimum of 1500 copies since its appearance on the Canadian market.

Hence, on the basis of the above investigations, it was not possible to satisfactorily establish the degree of popularity of these books within North America.

However, of the five selected popular books, P-5 has undergone three editions, and P-4 and P-1 are in their sixth and ninth printings, respectively. Hence one may at least assume a tradition of popular dissemination for these books. The remaining two books, P-2 and P-3, are still in their first printing.

Thus, largely on the basis of personal communication with 13 North American booksellers, and on the printing histories of four of the five selected books, an assumption has been made that the popular home medical books selected for this investigation enjoy at least a moderate degree of popular dissemination within North America.

4.   THE HISTORICAL CONTEXT: 'GENEALOGIES' OF THE SELECTED BOOKS

a.   *Texbooks of medicine*[8]

For those few Americans trained in medicine in the late eighteenth and early nineteenth centuries, access to current medical opinion was obtained primarily through American editions of books written by British and continental European physicians and scientists.[9] Only toward the middle of the nineteenth century did the United States start producing its own group of qualified textbook writers.[10] According to Harvey and McKusick,[11] the textbook of medicine most widely used toward the end of the nineteenth century (not only in North America, but in the entire English-speaking world) was Sir Thomas Watson's *Practice,* published in Britain in 1843.

In 1890 Dr. William Osler, distressed by what he considered to be the paucity of textbooks in medicine by American authors, and openly critical of the examples currently available, embarked upon the task of writing *The Principles and Practice of Medicine.*[12] Published in 1892, this work created a major prototype for all subsequent North American textbooks of medicine. Remarkable for its readable style,[13] its comprehensiveness in covering all aspects of the field, and its focus upon clinical problems rather than upon specific disease entities, this single-authored work became one of the most important national and international[14] sources for study throughout Osler's authorship (until 1914) as well as during its subsequent editorship by Thomas McCrae (until 1935) and Henry Christian (until 1947). This sixteenth edition in 1947 marked the end of the book's single-author tradition. Following a hiatus of 21 years, a group of Johns Hopkins faculty members took up the task of producing a seventeenth edition, continuing to give precedence, as Osler had done before them, to clinical problems rather than disease entities. Since the resumption of its publication in 1968, the chief editor of this textbook (for its seventeenth, eighteenth, and nineteenth editions) has been Abner McGehee Harvey.[15]

A second major influence in the field of North American textbook writing emerged in 1927. At that time, Russell Cecil was a young private practitioner in New York whose background had included academic medicine at the Rockefeller Institute and Bellevue. Acting upon his conviction that, given the growth and diversification of knowledge in internal medicine, textbooks in this subject should be multi-authored, rather than authored by a single person, Cecil wrote to prominent specialists in the field, requesting, and subsequently gaining, their expert contributions.[16] This cooperative effort resulted in the publication, in 1928, of the first edition of *Textbook of Medicine by American Authors*.[17] Cecil continued as the single editor of this multi-authored book up to, and including, the publication of its seventh edition in 1947. At this time, the phrase "by American Authors" had been dropped, its title appearing simply as *Textbook of Medicine*. Coedited by Robert Loeb and others for its eighth edition in 1951, the book retained its shortened title in all subsequent editions, with the exception of the eleventh, twelfth, and thirteenth editions, in which it was entitled the *Cecil-Loeb Textbook of Medicine*. Although the names of Cecil and Loeb no longer appear in the title, the present fourteenth edition of *Textbook of Medicine*, edited by Paul Beeson and Walsh McDermott,[18] is dedicated to their memory.

A third challenger to the field of textbook writing, whose innovative work exerted considerable influence, was Tinsley Harrison. A graduate of Johns Hopkins University in 1922, Harrison and a group of associate editors whose medical training had been deeply rooted in the basic sciences, decided in the late 1940s to create a textbook[19] in which issues of clinical medicine would be closely informed by the preclinical sciences:

They emphasized an approach that developed 'not only from the standpoint of disorders of structure, but also by way of abnormal physiology, chemistry, and disturbed psychology' . . . The modern ideal of clinical teaching holds that the classical approach, with primary emphasis on specific diseases, is inadequate, and that the student or practitioner cannot be expected to recognize disease in its various manifestations and to manage it intelligently unless he also understands the basic mechanism of its cardinal manifestations.[20]

The first edition of this work, entitled *Principles of Internal Medicine*,[21] appeared in 1950. Its current editor, George W. Thorn, was involved in that first edition.[22] Although Harrison did not serve as editor after the fifth edition in 1966, the current eighth edition now bears his name, viz. *Harrison's Principles of Internal Medicine*.

According to Bogdonoff, the number of dissimilarities that existed amongst the early editions of the three textbooks indicated above have, over the years, been greatly reduced:

The emphasis of the relevance of basic science to an understanding of clinical medicine has changed all textbooks of medicine during the past half century. . . . Thus, the three major American textbooks—Harrison, Beeson-

McDermott and Osler-Hopkins—are all essentially successful amalgamations of the basic sciences and descriptions of disease. Though the format may be somewhat different among them [the most notable difference, in the editions selected for this study, being the unique organization of the contents of T-1], there is a remarkable similarity in content among the three. There are some differences in details, but one can refer to any one of these books and come away with a satisfactory precis of process and entity for almost all of internal medicine.[23]

The state of affairs which Bogdonoff describes above, however, is not duplicated in the five popular books selected for this study, amongst which the reader will note that individual differences, both in form as well as in content, are far more marked than in the selected textbooks. The following brief review of the early history of these popular books helps to account for at least some of these dissimilarities.

b.   *Popular home medical books*

In a chapter entitled 'From Buchan to Fishbein: The Literature of Domestic Medicine',[24] John B. Blake provides an excellent historical review of what he calls 'household medical books'.

Acknowledging that 'popular medicine is ancient history', and that 'guides for self-treatment were neither new in the nineteenth century nor specifically American',[25] Blake suggests two eighteenth century British works which might reasonably be accepted as the key sources of two quite radically different 'streams' of domestic medical literature subsequently appearing in North America throughout the nineteenth and twentieth centuries. These two works are: William Buchan's *Domestic Medicine,* first published in Edinburgh in 1769,[26] and John Wesley's *Primitive Physick,* first published in London in 1747.[27]

Domestic books in the 'Buchan tradition' characteristically were claimed to be intended for persons who were living in remote areas, or were at sea in a ship, or were plantation owners who wished to treat their slaves.[28] Mostly written by doctors, these books routinely provided instruction on the prevention of illness and on the treatment of certain emergencies. They tended, implicitly or explicitly, to emphasize and reinforce the doctor's role in matters pertaining to health and disease. For example, one book belonging to this tradition expressed the view that 'it was much better for physicians to practice in families that knew something about medicine. They would be more likely to call the physician promptly when sick and to follow his instructions'.[29]

Within the earlier phase of the 'Buchan tradition', Blake locates the following six works:

1. William Buchan, *Domestic Medicine: or, the Family Physician* (Philadelphia: R. Aitken, 1771).
2. Anthony A. Benezet, *The Family Physician; Comprising Rules for the Prevention and Cure of Diseases; Calculated Particularly for the Inhabitants of the Western Country, and for Those Who Navigate its Waters* (Cincinnati: W.H. Woodward, 1826).
3. Thomas Ewell, *American Family Physician: Detailing Important Means of Preserving Health, from Infancy to Old Age* (Georgetown, D.C.: J. Thomas, 1824).
4. Thomas W. Ruble, *The American Medical Guide for the Use of Families* (Richmond, Ky.: E. Harris, 1810).
5. Thomas Cooper, *A Treatise of Domestic Medicine* (Reading, Pa.: G. Getz, 1824).
6. William Matthews, *A Treatise on Domestic Medicne* (sic) *and Kindred Subjects: Embracing Anatomical and Physiological Sketches of the Human Body* (Indianapolis: J.D. Defrees, 1848).

According to Blake, books belonging to a later phase of the 'Buchan tradition' had a somewhat different editorial emphasis. Not only was there a 'duty to enlighten the public, particularly on the means to avoid disease', but also to disseminate 'knowledge for its own sake'.[30] One representative author of this later tradition, George M. Beard, argued that 'the habit of looking at things from a scientific point of view was necessary if the country was to solve its many social and political problems'.[31] By this token, he attacked 'quacks . . . charlatans . . . (and) food faddists . . . for their erroneous and unscientific views'.[32]

As representative of this later phase of the 'Buchan tradition', Blake cites the following four books:

1. George M. Beard, *Our Home Physician: A New and Popular Guide to the Art of Preserving Health and Treating Disease* (New York: E.B. Treat, 1869).
2. Frederick A. Castle, ed., *Wood's Household Practice of Medicine, Hygiene and Surgery* (New York: W. Wood, 1880).
3. *The Home Medical Library* (New York: Review of Reviews Co., 1907).
4. Morris Fishbein, *Modern Home Medical Adviser; Your Health and How to Preserve It* (Garden City, N.Y.: Doubleday, Doran, 1935).

In contrast to the 'Buchan tradition', domestic books in the 'Wesley tradition' were typically hostile to doctors, to their methods of dealing with illness, and (not infrequently) to the size of their fees. Such books characteristically promoted 'common sense' remedies along with the notion of self-help, often with an underlying appeal to thrift:

Originally, according to Wesley, cures were empirical discoveries passed down from father to son, suited to the climate and available natural products of a particular region. But then men began to inquire into the causes of things. Discarding 'experiment' and simple medicines, they began to prescribe according to theory, and physic became an abstruse science out of the reach of ordinary men. When physicians found that this raised their status and enhanced their profits, they designedly increased the number of exotic drugs and the mystery surrounding medicine, while branding as empirics those who knew only how to restore the sick to health. His book, Wesley wrote, would return medicine to its primitive simplicity, when there was no need for anatomy or natural philosophy, but only the knowledge that 'Such a Medicine removes such a Pain'. Thus one could have a physician always in the home to prescribe without fee, and multitudes could be saved from pining away in sickness and pain through the ignorance or knavery of physicians.[33]

Blake identifies the following works as belonging to this tradition:

1. John Wesley, *Primitive Physick: or, an Easy and Natural Method of Curing Most Diseases*, 12th ed. (Philadelphia: A. Steuart, 1764).
2. Samuel North, *The Family Physician and Guide to Health, Together with Some Remarks on Surgery* (Waterloo, N.Y.: William Child, 1830).
3. Daniel H. Whitney, *The Family Physician and Guide to Health* (Penn-Yan, N.Y.: H. Gilbert, 1833).
4. John C. Gunn, *Gunn's Domestic Medicine, or Poor Man's Friend, in the Hours of Affliction, Pain and Sickness*, 4th ed. (Madisonville: Henderson and Johnston, 1834).
5. A.G. Goodlett, *The Family Physician, or Every Man's Companion* (Nashville, Tenn.: Smith and Nesbit, 1838).

As constituting a possible third 'stream' of American domestic medical books, Blake identifies another group of works which, while they did not attack the medical profession (as did those in the 'Wesley tradition'), tended instead to ignore it. Such books were in the format of recipes, 'often intermingling those for the cure of various diseases with various household receipts and farriery'.[34] Such recipes 'continued popular for years to come, not only in books but also in almanacs, newspapers, and similar forms of popular literature'.[35]

As belonging to this group (by virtue of their format), Blake cites the following works:

1. Lewis Merlin, *The Treasure of Health* (Philadelphia, 1819).
2. William Buchan, *Every Man His Own Doctor; or A Treatise on the Prevention and Cure of Diseases, by Regimen and Simple Medicines* (New Haven: N. Whiting, 1816).
3. Josiah Richardson, compiler, *The New-England Farrier, and Family Physician* (Exeter: J. Richardson, 1828).

Although the books which have been selected for this study fall, for the most part, within the 'Buchan tradition',[36] nevertheless, the occasional vestigial trace of an influence from the 'Wesley tradition' and from the 'recipe tradition' may still be seen amongst the various examples of material which (in subsequent sections) will be cited from the five popular books.

Finally, while it is evident from this brief historical review that both textbooks of medicine and popular home medical books can claim long historical traditions, it is further evident (see Graph 1 and Appendix A) that the three selected textbooks have had longer individual histories than is the case of the five popular books.

In concluding this section, it is important to note that the past two decades have seen the rise of a kind of medical literature whose authors and editors declare themselves to be in opposition to the tenets of conventional medicine. Since most of these books present arguments against the application of certain diagnostic and therapeutic technologies (including chemotherapy) in health care, they may perhaps best be described as 'counter-technological'. Included in this group would be the following':

1. Edward Bauman, et al., *The Holistic Health Handbook: A Tool for Attaining Wholeness of Body, Mind and Spirit* (Berkeley, Ca.: And/Or Press, 1978).
2. Brian Inglis, *The Case for Unorthodox Medicine* (New York: Putnam, 1969).
3. Dr. J.M. Jussawalla, *Healing From Within: A Treatise on the Philosophy and Theory of Nature Cure* (Bombay: Manaktalas, 1966).
4. Jack La Patra, *Healing: The Coming Revolution in Holistic Medicine* (New York: McGraw-Hill, 1978).
5. Donald Law, *A Guide to Alternative Medicine* (Garden City, N.Y.: Dolphin - Doubleday, 1976).
6. Chris Popenoe, *Wellness* (Washington: YES! Inc., 1977).
7. Julius A. Roth, *Health Purifiers and their Enemies* (New York: Prodist, 1977).

Graph 1. *'Genealogies' of books of medical instruction*

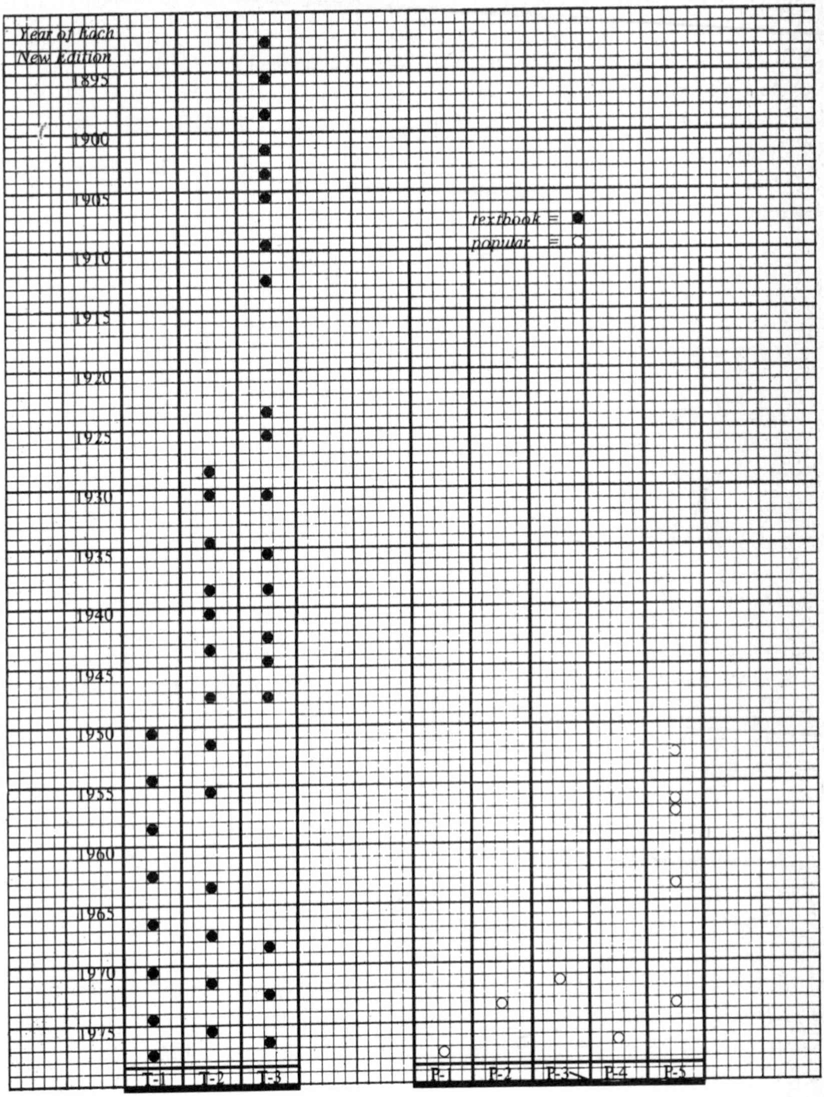

8. Donald A. Tubesing, *Wholistic Health* (New York: Human Sciences Press, 1979).
9. Wallis Roy and Peter Morley, eds., *Marginal Medicine* (London: Peter Owen, 1976).

5.   THE CRITICAL CONTEXT:[37] CRITICAL REVIEWS OF SELECTED BOOKS

The appearance of a new book in print (or of a new edition of an existing book) usually provokes the subsequent appearance of a book review.[38] On one level, a book review may be seen as a cultural 'feedback mechanism', wherein a reviewer (presumably selected by his employers as a kind of ideally-discriminating and disinterested reader) may criticize, praise, or otherwise interpret the form and contents of a particular book to the readership of whichever print vehicle carries that review (be it a newspaper, a journal, or a magazine). The printed review, in its turn, frequently provokes responses from the readers, some of whose 'letters to the editor' may come to be printed. Not infrequently, a book review has been known to provoke a response even from the author himself. In short, the institution of the printed book review permits the possibility of a dialogue in print between the reviewer and the reader, the reviewer and the author, and even the author and the reader, any or all of which may influence the author of the reviewed book with respect to his future writing efforts.

In the special case of those who write critiques of medical textbooks, one would expect that the minimal requirements in the hiring of a person for such a task are that (a) he has studied medicine (and, ideally, has practised it as well), and (b) he has a high degree of 'fluency' in the use of contemporary scientific medical English.

Moreover, with respect to those who read such critiques (which, in all discovered examples, are printed exclusively in journals addressed to members of the medical or paramedical professions), it is highly probable that they, too, have a level of background knowledge and skill in the use of scientific medical language which at least approximate that of the textbook author.

Let us now assume that both textbooks and popular books will express certain theories pertaining to the field of medicine. According to Popper, '. . . the criterion of the scientific theory is its falsifiability, or refutability, or testability'.[39] For a theory to be refutable, however, it must be stated in language which is rigorously standardized, such that it is characteristically formal (rather than informal or colloquial), systematic (rather than erratic), precise (rather than vague), and nonambiguous (rather than open to many different kinds of interpretation). Moreover, for such a theory to be successfully refuted, the would-be refuter must have an adequate understanding of the consequences of that theory. This cannot be the case, however, if he lacks sufficient background knowledge in the basic sciences which inform medical theories.

If the reader will turn for a moment to Table 1 and to Appendix B, it will be evident that reviews of textbooks of medicine, typically (a) are written by doctors, and (b) appear in journals addressed to members of the medical or paramedical professions. Conversely, reviews of popular home medical books, typically (a) are not written by doctors, and (b) appear only in newspapers, magazines, or library review journals, none of which can claim a majority readership informed in the medical sciences. Therefore it is clear that the institution of the medical journal book review helps to guarantee informed 'feedback' to the author of a reviewed textbook, and thereby increases the probability that, on the basis of such criticism, he may revise his theories in subsequent editions of that textbook. In contrast, although a nonmedical person (be he the book reviewer or the reader of the book review) may also elect to challenge a theory which a popular author has put forth in his book, he can do so only in a very general manner, such that there will be little if any influence upon that author with respect to any subsequent revision of that theory for future editions of that book.

NOTES

1. With respect to this criterion, see Part Two, Section II: 3(c) (ii).
2. The term 'current' will be defined here as 'having appeared in a new or revised edition within the past ten years' (i.e. not before 1970).
3. With respect to this criterion, see Part One, Section II: 2 above.
4. With respect to this criterion, see Part One, Section II: 3 above.
5. Throughout this investigation, reference to the selected books will be made by means of an abbreviated 'code'. The number indicating the sequence in which the books have been listed above, preceded by the appropriate capital letter, will determine the code. Thus the three *t*extbooks of medicine will be coded as T-1, T-2, and T-3 respectively, while the five *p*opular home medical books will be coded as P-1, P-2, P-3, P4, and P-5 respectively.
6. The sequence of the three textbooks in Part A of the questionnaire was varied in the letters sent out in order to preclude the possibility that a fixed sequence might prejudice the results.
7. Morton D. Bogdonoff, 'Book reviews', *The New England Journal of Medicine* 301 (July 26, 1979): 220.
8. A brief summary of the histories of the three selected textbooks of medicine appears in Bogdonoff 1979: 220-222. Also, see Appendix A for 'genealogies' of the successive editions of each of these three books.
   For historical data pertaining to the publication of American medical textbooks,

Table 1.   *Distribution of book reviews of selected books of medical instruction*

(a)   Textbooks

T-1	T-2	T-3
Continuing Education for the Family Physician, July 1978, pp. 64-66. *Annals of Internal Medicine*, 1977, vol. 87, p. 129. *Medical Textbook Review*, Medical Sickness Annuity and Life Assurance Society Ltd., London, pp. 31-32.	*Continuing Education for the Family Physician*, July 1978, pp. 64-66. *Annals of Internal Medicine*, 1976, vol. 84, pp. 109-110. *Medical Textbook Review*, Medical Sickness Annuity and Life Assurance Society Ltd., London, p. 31.	*Continuing Education for the Family Physician*, July 1978, p. 66. *Annals of Internal Medicine*, 1976, vol. 85, pp. 699-700. *Medical Textbook Review*, Medical Sickness Annuity and Life Assurance Society Ltd., London, pp. 31-32.
	Delaware Medical Journal, May 1976, vol. 48, no. 1, p. 302. *Dermatology*, Nov. 1976, p. 702. *Plastic and Reconstructive Surgery*, Oct. 1976, p. 498. *Unlisted Drugs*, July 1976, vol. 28, no. 7, p. 124. *Tic*, Oct. 1976, p. 6. *The Lancet*, Feb. 7, 1976, p. 285.	*Delaware Medical Journal*, Mar. 1978, vol. 50, no. 3, p. 172. *Chest*, May 1977, vol. 71, p. 28.

contd.

Table 1 (*contd.*)

(b) Popular books

P-1 and *P-2*

Unable to locate.

P-3

Kirkus Reviews, vol. 39, July 1971.
Science Books, American Association for the Advancement of Science, vol. 8, no. 1, May, 1972.
Library Journal, vol. 96, no. 13, July, 1971.
Choice, Association of College and Research Libraries, American Library Assocaition, vol. 8, no. 10, Dec., 1971.

P-4

Stanley News and Press, Albermarle, N.C., July 27, 1976.
Choice, December, 1976.
Baltimore, Md., *Morning Sun*, Oct. 31, 1977.
American Reference Book Annual, 1977.
San Francisco Review of Books, Nov. 1976.
Independent Press, Jan. 26, 1977.
Garden City, N.Y. *Newsday*, June 20, 1977.
Jackson, Tenn., *Sun*, July 11, 1976.
Independent Review Service, Baltimore, Md. Dec. 14, 1976.
Daily Record, Morris County, N.J., Aug. 8, 1976.
San Francisco, Calif., *Chronicle*, July 26, 1976.

P-5

American Reference Book Annual, 1975, ed. by Bohdan S. Wynar. Littleton: Libraries Unlimited, 1975.

see Barbara Coe Johnson, 'Medical book publishing', *Library Trends* 7 (July, 1958): 210-219; also Gertrude L. Annan, 'Medical Americana', *Journal of the American Medical Association* 192 (1965): 139-144. Additional data on this subject is available as well in two works dealing with the history of American companies which publish medical textbooks, i.e. *Philadelphia's Publishers and Printers: An Informal History*, ed. by Kenneth Bussy (Philadelphia: Philadelphia Book Clinic, 1976) and Gerard R. Wolfe, 'The Appletons: Four generations of publishing in America' (Ph.D. dissertation, Union Graduate School, 1978).

For those interested in a comprehensive historical outline of medical books since antiquity, see J.L. Thornton, *Medical Books, Libraries and Collectors* (London: Andre Deutsch, 1966).

9. Gertrude L. Annan cites in particular the works of Baillie, Cadogan, Cheselden, Cullen, Denman, Hunter, and (Benjamin, Charles, and John) Bell (from Britain); and the translated works of Alibert, Bichat, Blumenbach, Corvisart, Haller, Larrey, Senec, and Tissot (from the Continent). Annan 1965: 142.

10. In Thomas E. Keys, 'Some American medical imprints of the nineteenth century', *Bulletin of the Medical Library Association* 45 (1957): 309-318, the first American medical textbook is cited as James Thacher, *American Modern Practice* (Boston: E. Read, 1817). Annan 1965: 142, cites as the American 'giants' of nineteenth century textbook writing the works of Beaumont, McDowell, Simms, Drake, Gross, Mott, Bowditch, Shattuck, and 'a host of others'.

11. Abner McGehee Harvey and Victor A. McKusick, eds., *Osler's Textbook Revisited* (New York: Appleton-Century-Crofts, 1967), p. 1.

12. Sir William Osler, born in Bond Head, Ontario in 1849, was Professor of the Institute of Medicine at McGill University from 1874 until 1884, then was Professor of Clinical Medicine at the University of Pennsylvania from 1884 to 1887. While Professor of Medicine at the Johns Hopkins University and Physician-in-Chief of the newly-opened (1889) Johns Hopkins Hospital, Osler devoted two years (from 1890 to 1892) to the writing of *The Principles and Practice of Medicine*. Its current 'descendent', T-3, is one of the three books investigated in this study. For an interesting account of the circumstances under which Osler first published his famous work, see Harvey and McKusick 1967: 1-12. See also Wolfe 1978: 112-121.

13. 'It has been said that in his textbook, Olser "succeeded in making a scientific treatise literature" '. Harvey and McKusick 1967: 4.

14. 'Cushing remarked: "Someone, some day, could well write a volume devoted to the study of the successive editions of this famous work which continues to exercise an enormous influence on students of medicine—even beyond English-reading countries through its many translations" (French, 1908; German, 1909; Chinese, 1910 and 1921, and Spanish, 1915)'. Harvey and McKusick 1967: 4-5.

15. See Appendix C for biographical data on current editors.

16. Bogdonoff 1979: 220.

17. T-2, its 'descendant', is one of the three textbooks investigated in this study.

18. See Appendix C for biographical data on current editors.

19. See Appendix G for historical data.

20. Bogdonoff 1979: 220.

21. T-1, its 'descendant', is one of the three textbooks investigated in this study.

22. See Appendix C for biographical data on current editors.

23. Bogdonoff 1979: 220.

24. Guenter B. Risse et al., eds., *Medicine Without Doctors* (New York: Science History Publications, 1977), pp. 11-29.

25. Risse et al. 1977: 27.
26. According to Annan 1965: 141, this book underwent more than 30 American editions between 1771 and 1815, having been revised 'according to the diseases and climate of the United States'.
27. This book was subsequently reprinted in Philadelphia in 1764 and continued in popularity in America until well into the nineteenth century. Blake, 'From Buchan to Fishbein', in Risse et al. 1977: 18.
28. Risse et al. 1977: 16.
29. Risse et al. 1977: 16.
30. Risse et al. 1977: 27.
31. Risse et al. 1977: 27.
32. Risse et al. 1977: 27-28.
33. Risse et al. 1977: 18-19.
34. Blake notes that material of this type was frequently included in eighteenth century cookbooks. He also points out that Wesley's *Primitive Physick* was written in this kind of format. Risse et al. 1977: 25.
35. Risse et al. 1977: 26.
36. This may be confirmed by the fact that all five popular books contain sentences which reinforce, to the reader, the importance of the doctor's role in the treatment of disease. See Supplement A-5.
37. Concerning the notion of a 'critical context' or of a 'critical tradition', the reader is referred to the works of Karl R. Popper, especially *Objective Knowledge: An Evolutionary Approach* (London: Oxford University Press, 1972) and *Conjectures and Refutations: The Growth of Scientific Knowledge* (New York: Harper and Row, 1965).
38. See Table 1 for a list of the locations of book reviews, and Appendix B for the actual reviews. The reviews in Appendix B were obtained following an extensive library search in medical journals and reviewing journals. Also, some publishers of the selected books cooperated, either through sending copies of reviews of their books, or by indicating their locations. As is evident from Table 1, the writer was unable to locate book reviews for either P-1 or P-2.
39. Popper 1965: 37.

PART TWO

A Semiotic Comparison of Textbooks of Medicine and Popular Home Medical Books

Explanation of Technical Terms
and Methods of Analysis

1. *Semiotics*

The term 'semiotics' is defined as that field of theoretical and applied knowledge which addresses itself to the systematic study of signs and the signifying process (semiosis).[1] Thus the title of this study indicates that two groups of books, textbooks of medicine and popular home medical books, are to be compared with respect to the properties of their constituent signs.

2. *Linguistics*

'Linguistics may be defined as the scientific study of language' . . . Semiotics, on the other hand, sometimes also called semiology, does not study only human or verbal language, it also studies animal languages and all systems of communication, natural or artificial, employed by men, animals, and real or ideal machines. From these two definitions, it follows that the subject-matter of linguistics forms only a part of the subject-matter of semiotics.[2]

3. *Linguistic properties*

The major focus of this study will be on linguistic rather than nonlinguistic signs (such as illustrations).[3] Linguistic signs in textbooks and popular books will be compared in terms of the following linguistic properties:
(a) phonological - the sound properties of language[4] (e.g. alliteration and syllabification)
(b) grammatical - grammatical categories (e.g. pronouns, compound nouns, etc.)
  - syntax (the manner of combining words into phrases, sentences, etc.)

(c) semantic   - the meaning and/or scope of certain words or groups of words

(d) pragmatic   - the contextual circumstances impinging upon the selection or interpretation of words or groups of words (e.g. the intention of the author, the effect upon the reader, etc.).[5]

Analyses of such properties as are described above have been applied to segments of the eight selected books.

4. Segments

A segment is defined as any conventionally-differentiated portion of a book which contributes to its major formal design. Each book consists of three segments: (a) the Table of Contents; (b) the Text; and (c) the Paratext. Since (a) is self-explanatory, only (b) and (c) will be defined below:

The term 'Text' will be strictly reserved for that portion of a book which extends from the beginning of the first chapter up to the end of the final chapter. With the exception of the Table of Contents (which constitutes a segment in and of itself), all additional portions of the book which either precede or follow the Text (such as the Title Page, the List of Contributing Authors, the Preface, the Introduction, the Index, the Appendix, and so on) will be said to constitute the Paratext.

In order to arrive at a comprehensive comparison of the semiotic properties of the selected books, all three segments have been investigated in this study.

5. Elements

The three segments of the book, indicated above, are in turn composed of three different kinds of elements: (a) discursive, (b) nondiscursive, and (c) tabular.

(a)   Discursive elements consist of sequences of sentences, examples of which are paragraphs (or parts of paragraphs) and chapters. These sentences are composed of linguistic signs drawn primarily from natural language, but also include signs drawn from certain artificial languages (e.g. mathematics).

Individual words will be referred to either as 'lexical items' or else as 'terms'. Also, such phrases as 'multiple sclerosis' and 'muscular dystrophy' will be referred to as 'terms'.

The expression 'main lexical item' will be taken to mean any word belonging to any of the grammatical categories, with the exceptions of prepositions, definite and indefinite articles, and conjunctions.

(b)   Nondiscursive elements, in contrast to discursive elements, are characteristically not part of a coherent discourse. Examples include bibliographical references, citations, index items, names of contributing authors, the recto and verso of pages, illustrations (e.g. photographs, tables, graphs), and so on. Thus, nondiscursive elements include both linguistic and nonlinguistic signs.[6]

(c)   Tabular elements constitute the third kind of element characteristic of these books, and are exemplified by (1) the set of headings of which the Table of Contents of each book is composed, and (2) the set of bold-type headings typically interspersed throughout each Disease Description.

6.   Selected Headings

The set of major headings constituting the Table of Contents will be designated 'Selected Headings'.[7]

7.   Schemata

The set of bold-type headings typically interspersed throughout each Disease Description will be referred to as a 'Schema' (plural 'Schemata').

8.   Disease Descriptions

Any self-contained set of descriptive statements subsumed under the name of a particular disease will be called a 'Disease Description'.[8]

9.   Terms for aberrant states, or for indicators of aberrant states

The term 'aberrant state' has been selected by the writer as a broad umbrella term with which to designate any physical, mental, and, in some cases, social state considered to be abnormal or undersirable in light of current expectations, norms, or 'goals' based upon a hypothesized optimal function, appearance, sensation, or behavior of the human organism.[9]

The term 'indicator of aberrant state' will be used to refer to any phenomenon that is assumed to be a sign, symptom, or manifestation of some aberrant state.

Both of these terms, 'aberrant state' and 'indicator of aberrant state',[10] may, on the basis of their degree of generality, be divided into two types: Type One and Type Two.

Type One Terms: These include terms which refer in a nonspecific way either to aberrant states (e.g. the terms 'disease', 'disorder', 'ailment') or else to indicators of aberrant states (e.g. the terms 'symptom', 'sign', 'manifestation', or 'complaint').

Type Two Terms: These include terms which refer either to relatively restricted subclasses of aberrant states (e.g. 'asthma', 'Parkinson's disease', and 'diverticulitis') or to relatively specific indicators of aberrant states (e.g. 'cough', 'headache', 'hematuria', etc.). The former group of terms are frequently used as diagnostic labels; the latter group as names of symptoms or signs.

10. *Sentences of pragmatic instruction*

A special group of sentences has been identified, examples of which appear in all of the selected books. These sentences are characterized by the fact that they are intended to influence the reader in carrying out certain practical actions, that is to say, to provoke pragmatic consequences. Hence they have been named 'sentences of pragmatic instruction', of which two types have been noted: 'imperious' and 'nonimperious'. The imperious type typically affords the reader no option in the carrying out of the instruction. They include imperative sentences (i.e. commands), as well as normative sentences. Non-imperious sentences, by contrast, are less 'verbally coercive', and include 'advisory' sentences (e.g. 'It is suggested that x be done'), as well as 'exemplary' sentences (e.g. 'In situation x, y is done'). These sentences will be discussed in greater detail in Supplement A-2, and numerous examples will be given to demonstrate the above distinctions.

11. *Methods of semiotic analysis described*

In the process of establishing how textbooks of medicine differ semiotically from popular home medical books, essentially six kinds of analytic methods have been applied to the segments of the selected books. These include the following:

(a)   Sentential Analyses: the relative distribution of sentences identified according to certain grammatical, semantic, and pragmatic properties has been measured in the eight Disease Descriptions of diabetes mellitus.

(b)   Lexical Analyses: the relative distribution of lexical items displaying certain grammatical, semantic, and phonological properties has been measured, both in Disease Descriptions of diabetes mellitus, as well as in Selected Headings.

(c)   Rhetorical Analyses: the presence has been noted of various rhetorical devices (such as popular metaphors, alliteration, hyperbole, cliches, testimonials, etc.) found exclusively in the Disease Descriptions of the popular books. Such devices contribute towards the colloquial style which characterizes these books as a group. Numerous examples are to be found in Supplement A-3.

(d)   Quantifications of Certain Nondiscursive Elements: Such quantifications have yielded significant values which were subsequently compared in the two groups of books (values such as the reference-to-page ratio, the illustration-to-page ratio, and the author-to-page ratio).

(e)   Mapping Methods Involving Tabular Elements: Two kinds of tabular elements have already been identified: Selected Headings and Schemata (see Section I: 5 [c] above). Comparing such tabular elements from book to book presented a considerable methodological challenge, owing to their broad and diverse range of linguistic properties. This problem was met by means of recruiting two 'external standards' in relation to which the data could be 'standardized' prior to being cross-compared. In the case of the Selected Headings, the standard was provided by the 17 'Categories' of the 'List of Three-digit Categories',[11] whereas in the case of the Schemata, the standard was provided by the 32 chapter headings of *Joslin's Diabetes Mellitus.*[12] In both cases, certain lexical items belonging to the headings in question were 'mapped' upon certain other lexical items belonging to the external standard, on the basis of there being some kind of semantic correlation between them. This procedure will be described in greater detail in Section II: 1(d), and 2(c) which follow.

(f)   Questionnaires and Library Searches: In order to discover some of the social, historical, and critical contexts in which the selected books are involved, data was gathered in a number of ways: (i) personal communication with the editors;[13] (ii) a postal questionnaire sent to 136 North American medical school libraries; (iii) library searches for critical reviews, for biographical data on the authors or editors, and for historical data relating to the history of books of medical instruction in general, and to the 'genealogy' of each book in particular.

The methods indicated above have been described in greater detail in the course of their respective applications to the various elements of the selected books.

12. *Rationale underlying selection of elements for analysis*

According to the methods of analysis outlined in the previous section, an investigation has been made of the three kinds of semiotic elements earlier indicated: discursive, nondiscursive, and tabular. Opposite the name of each element, the rationale for its analysis will be made clear.

A.   *Nondiscursive elements*

Type of element quantified	*Rationale for selection*
(i) Pages	To determine if difference in length as established by the number of pages in the Text is a distinguishing feature between textbooks of medicine and popular home medical books.
(ii) Bibliographical References or Citations	To determine if the reference-to-page ratio is a distinguishing feature.[14]
(iii) Illustrations (photographs, tables, graphs, etc.)	To determine if the illustration-to-page ratio is a distinguishing feature.
(iv) Authors and their Academic Status (from List of Contributing Authors)	To determine if the author-to-page-ratio is a distinguishing feature. Also, to determine whether the academic status of the authors and editors constitutes a distinguishing feature.
(v) Number of Editions (from the verso of the Title Page)	To determine if (a) the number of editions the book has undergone, and (b) the rate of appearance of new editions, are distinguishing features.
(vi) Number of Translations (from the verso of the Title Page)	To determine if the number of languages into which the books have been translated is a distinguishing feature.
(vii) Other Miscellaneous Elements from the Paratext (such as Dedications, Lists of Other Books by the same author, Warnings regarding drug therapy administration, etc.)	To determine if the presence or absence of any of these miscellaneous elements is a distinguishing feature.

B.   *Discursive elements*

Type of Element Quantified	Rationale for Selection
(i) Discursive Material under such Headings as 'Preface', 'Introduction', 'Foreword', etc.	To determine if difference in editorial stance is a distinguishing feature, the 'editorial stance' being derived from statements expressing particular attitudes vis-à-vis: (a) doctors, (b) the readers, and (c) the perceived function of the book.
(ii) Discursive Material from the Text, Identified as a Disease Description (descriptions of the disease diabetes mellitus).	To determine how Disease Descriptions in textbooks differ from those in popular books with respect to form and contents.

C.   *Tabular elements*

(i)   Table of Contents: Selected Headings[15]

(i)   To establish which topics from the broad domain of medicine have been included and excluded (vis-à-vis the 'List of Three-digit Categories' in the *Manual*), for the purpose of determining whether there are significant differences between textbooks of medicine and popular home medical books with respect to their scope.

(ii) To compare the linguistic properties of the lexical items which constitute the headings, for the purpose of determining whether they differ significantly in textbooks of medicine as compared with popular books. (It has been assumed by the writer that the linguistic properties of these headings are very likely to be representative of the properties of the lexical items dispersed throughout the Text.)

(iii) To identify three classes of lexical items in Selected Headings: Class T (exclusive to textbooks), Class P (exclusive to popular books), Class T ∩ P (common to both).

Type of Element Quantified	*Rationale for Selection*
(ii) Schema of a Particular Disease Description: Diabetes Mellitus	To establish which aspects of a topic (i.e. of the topic 'diabetes mellitus') have been included or excluded (vis-à-vis the 32 chapter headings of *Joslin's*), for the purpose of discovering whether textbook descriptions differ from popular descriptions in terms of the concepts they emphasize.

NOTES

1. For a historical outline of the development of various theories of signs, the reader is referred to ' "Semiotics" and its congeners' in Sebeok, *Studies in Semiotics: Contributions to the Doctrine of Signs* (Bloomington: Indiana University Press, 1976), pp. 47-58.
2. Tullio de Mauro, 'The link with linguistics', in *The Tell-Tale Sign*, ed. Thomas A. Sebeok (Lisse, Netherlands: Peter de Ridder Press, 1975), p. 37.
3. However, certain nonlinguistic signs have been compared quantitatively in textbooks vs popular books.
4. John Lyons, *Introduction to Theoretical Linguistics* (London: Cambridge University Press, 1968), p. 54.
5. '. . . one may study the relations of signs to the objects to which signs are applicable. This relation will be called the semantical dimension of semiosis . . . The study of this dimension will be called *semantics*. Or the subject of study may be the relation of signs to interpreters . . . and the study of this dimension will be named *pragmatics* . . . Since all signs are potentially if not actually related to other signs, it is well to make a third dimension of semiosis . . . and the study of this dimension will be named *syntactics*'. (my emphasis). (Charles W. Morris, *Foundations of the Theory of Signs*, vol. 1, no. 1 (Chicago: University of Chicago Press, 1970), pp. 6-7.
6. Discursive elements are found mainly in the Text, but appear as well in the Preface, Introduction, or Appendix of the Paratext. Similarly, nondiscursive elements appear mainly in the Text (i.e. illustrations, citations, etc.) but may also be found in the Paratext (e.g. in the List of Contributing Authors).
7. In a few cases, and for reasons that will later be indicated, certain subheadings have been included in the Selected Headings as well.
8. The disease whose description will be investigated in this study is that of diabetes mellitus.
9. Ideally, the user of this term should specify the level of the 'system' which is assumed with respect to the goal or norm in question: whether physical, chemical, biological, psychological, or sociological. For example, malingering might be considered to constitute an aberrant state in an individual belonging to a society in which a disposition to work is assumed to be a sign of health, and its total absence, a sign of some disorder or disease. With respect to levels other than pyschological or

sociological, however, that individual might otherwise be considered to be in an optimal state of health. See Mario Bunge, *Scientific Research 1: The Search for System* (New York: Springer-Verlag, 1967), p. 24, with respect to his classification of the sciences.

10. Examples may be found in Supplements B-10 and B-11.

11. The 'List of Three-digit Categories' in World Health Organization, *Manual of the International Statistical Classification of Disease, Injuries, and Causes of Death.* Based on the recommendations of the Ninth Revision Conference, 1975, and adopted by the Twenty-ninth World Health Assembly (Geneva: World Health Organization, 1977), I, 1, hereafter cited as WHO *Manual.*

12. Alexander Marble et al., eds., *Joslin's Diabetes Mellitus* (Philadelphia: Lea and Febiger, 1971), pp. xi-xii, hereafter cited as *Joslin's.*

13. See Appendix G.

14. Throughout the remainder of this section, the term 'distinguishing feature' is to be understood as a feature which distinguishes between textbooks of medicine and popular home medical books.

15. Selected Headings are (with a few exceptions that will be later specified) identical with the major headings of a Table of Contents.

Semiotic Analyses of the Segments

1. THE TEXT[1]

a. *Its purpose*

In the case of each book, the Text is intended to educate and instruct the anticipated readers (whether 'lay' or 'professional') about selected aspects of the theory and practice of medicine in North America, for the purpose of teaching self-help, or of teaching the reader how to help others, or both. Editorial statements to this effect appear in the prefatory material of each Paratext (see Section II: 3 following). Moreover, a special group of sentences, identified as 'sentences of pragmatic instruction',[2] have been found to be common to the Texts of both textbooks of medicine and popular home medical books. These two factors, then, justify the subsumption of both groups of books under the designation 'books of medical instruction'.

b. *Its composition*

The Text is composed primarily of discursive elements, i.e. of sequences of sentences in natural language. These sentences either express, assume, or imply certain propositions pertaining to the theory and practice of medicine. All such propositions will be called 'medical statements'. Medical statements will be said to include all statements which have hitherto been formulated (or could in the future be formulated) about the nature, cause, prevention, treatment, or 'significance' of human disease (in the sense of 'moral', 'historical', or 'socioeconomic significance') and about the nature, promotion, maintenance, or 'significance' (as above) of human health. All such statements will be said to belong to the semantic domain[3] of Medicine.

c. *Disease Descriptions: Rationale for the selection of the disease, diabetes mellitus*

A characteristic feature of the Texts of books of medical instruction is the Disease Description, which is a self-contained set of medical statements subsumed under the name of a particular disease. A sample description has been selected for analysis on the assumption that it will indicate certain semiotic properties which may be claimed to be representative of the Text.

Descriptions of the disease, diabetes mellitus (three from the textbooks, and five from the popular home medical books), have been selected for the following reasons:

1. Diabetes mellitus, while constituting a well-circumscribed disease, embraces a wide number of manifestations involving numerous systems of the human organism. Hence, descriptions of this disease tend not only to be lengthy, but also, because they make use of a wide variety of explanatory strategies, they may be said to adequately exemplify the semiotic properties of the Text. Moreover, a description of this disease appears in every one of the eight selected books.

2. Diabetes has a high prevalence in North America,[4] which makes relevant a cross-textual comparison of descriptions of this disease appearing in North American books of medical instruction.

3. Diabetes is an ancient disease.[5] Hence, there exists a long historical tradition of recorded descriptions which could, at some future time, be evaluated in comparison with the present study.

d. *Comparison of Disease Descriptions: Textbook vs popular*

In this section, a number of Tables[6] will appear, indicating the distribution of certain semiotic properties found in the Disease Descriptions of diabetes mellitus. Frequent references will be made to these Tables in Part Three, as evidence bearing upon how textbooks of medicine and popular home medical books differ, both in their form as well as in their contents.

Method: All semiotic properties of Disease Descriptions which have been compared quantitatively from book to book have been actually counted, rather than having been estimated on the basis of a portion of the description. Given the highly uneven nature of the selected descriptions, the latter method would not have yielded as accurate a representation of the distribution of these properties.

In order to establish the number of sentences in each description, the actual number of sentences was tabulated. However, in estimating the number of words in each description, a ten-line sample was selected in each case, on the basis of which the average number of words per line was established. This number was then multiplied by the actual number of lines in each description. The results of these preliminary quantifications appear in Table 2.

While the writer is aware that eight Disease Descriptions of diabetes mellitus (one from each of the eight books) may be too small a sample from which to make statistical inferences with a high degree of accuracy, it was nevertheless felt that quantifications of the type that have been undertaken here are of intrinsic interest.

The semiotic properties of the eight selected Disease Descriptions will now be compared: (i) according to properties of sentences, (ii) according to properties of lexical items, (iii) according to other kinds of semiotic elements, and (iv) according to properties of their Schemata.

i.   *Properties of sentences*

The distribution has been determined of sentences identified according to the following properties: [a]   grammatical, [b] pragmatic, [c] semantic, [d] stylistic, and [e] 'special contents'.

Table 2.   *Numbers of sentences, words, and words per sentence in Disease Descriptions of diabetes mellitus*

(a) Textbooks					
No. of sentences		*No. of words*		*Words per sentence*	
T-1	667	T-1	14,938	T-1	22
T-2	660	T-2	18,762	T-2	28
T-3	855	T-3	19,768	T-3	23
Total	2182	Total	53,468		
Average	727	Average	17,823	Average	*24.3*

(b) Popular Books					
No. of sentences		*No. of words*		*Words per sentence*	
P-1	274	P-1	4,940	P-1	18
P-2	29	P-2	604	P-2	21
P-3	125	P-3	2,759	P-3	22
P-4	313	P-4	7,528	P-4	24
P-5	51	P-5	888	P-5	17
Total	792	Total	16,719		
Average	158	Average	3,344	Average	*20.4*

Graph 2. *Numbers of sentences, words, and words per sentence in Disease Descriptions of diabetes mellitus*

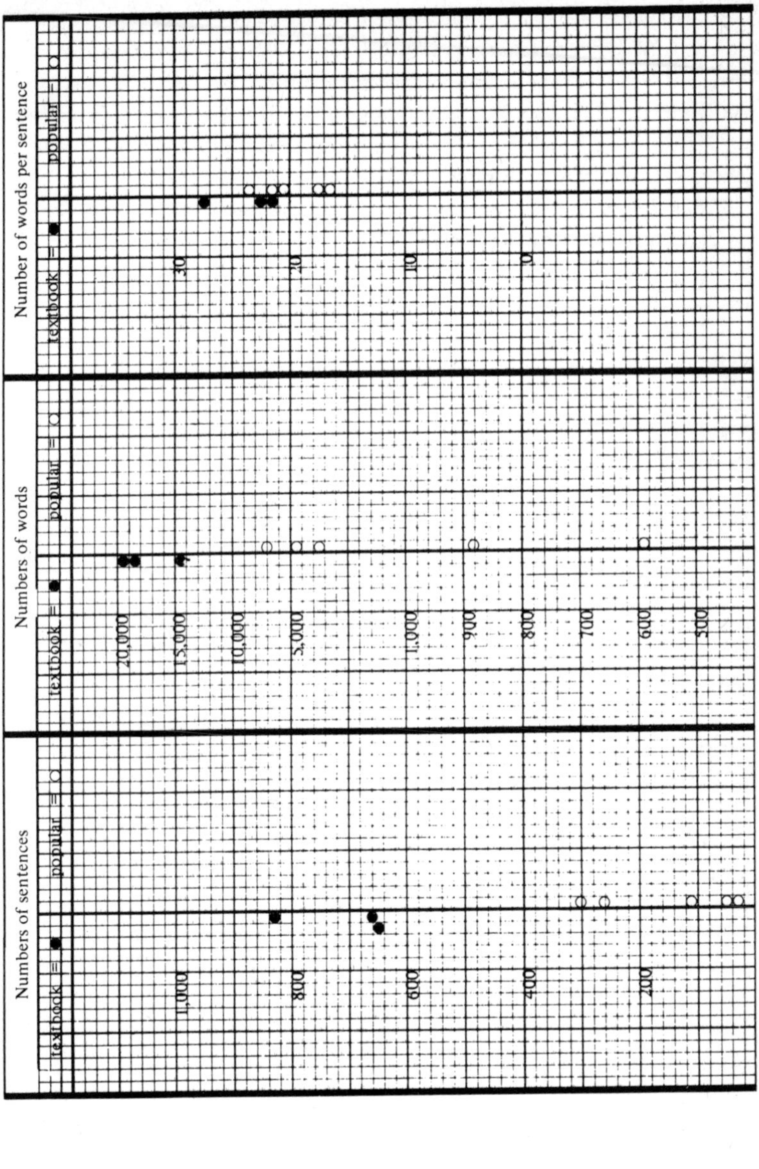

[a]   Grammatical Properties of Sentences: quantifications have been made of simple sentences as distinct from nonsimple sentences (i.e. compound, complex, and compound-complex types[7]) (see Table 3).

[b]   Pragmatic Properties of Sentences: quantifications have been made of sentences of pragmatic instruction: imperious vs nonimperious types (see Table 4, and for examples, see Supplement A-2).

[c]   Semantic Properties of Sentences: quantifications have been made of traditional sentence types, i.e. assertive, interrogative, imperative, and exclamatory[8] (see Table 5).

[d]   Stylistic Properties of Sentences: these include sentences constructed in a colloquial manner. Since they are exclusive to popular Disease Descriptions, they have not been quantified (see Supplement A-3 for examples).

[e]   Sentences with 'Special Contents': these are sentences which have been identified not on the basis of their formal properties, but rather on the basis of their special contents. These include [i] sentences which impart reassurance, hope, or optimism to the reader (see Supplement A-4 for examples), and [ii] sentences which reinforce, to the reader, the role of the doctor in the treatment of disease (see Supplement A-5 for examples).

The distribution of sentences classified according to [a], [b], and [c] above will now be demonstrated in Tables 3, 4, and 5, as well as in their companion Graphs. Since sentences classified according to [d] and [e] above occur only in popular books, no Tables appear for these items. However, as indicated above, they are exemplified in Supplement A.

ii.   *Properties of lexical items*

Lexical items in Disease Descriptions of diabetes mellitus have been investigated according to the following properties: [a] grammatical and [b] semantic.

[a]   Grammatical Properties of Lexical Items: quantifications have been made of:
   [i]   Interesentential markers of coherence.[9] See Table 6.
   [ii]   Personal pronouns.[10] See Table 7.
[b]   Semantic Properties of Lexical Items: quantifications have been made of:
   [i]   Terms naming biochemicals.[11] See Table 8.
   [ii]   Terms belonging to the semantic domain of food, diet, and dietary supplements. See Table 9.

Table 3. *Distribution in Disease Descriptions of sentence types: Simple vs nonsimple*

	T-1	T-2	T-3	Total	%[a]	P-1	P-2	P-3	P-4	P-5	Total	%[a]
Total no. of sentences in disease description	667	660	855	2,182		274	29	125	313	51	792	
Simple	362	321	474	1,157	53	145	7	57	156	22	387	49
%[b]	54	49	55			53	24	46	50	43		
Nonsimple	305	339	381	1,025	47	129	22	68	157	29	405	51
%[b]	46	51	45			47	76	54	50	57		

[a] Based on group totals of numbers of sentences in Disease Descriptions.
[b] Based on individual totals of numbers of sentences in Disease Descriptions (see Table 2).

Graph 3.

(a) *Simple sentences: individual percentages*

(b) *Nonsimple sentences: individual percentages*

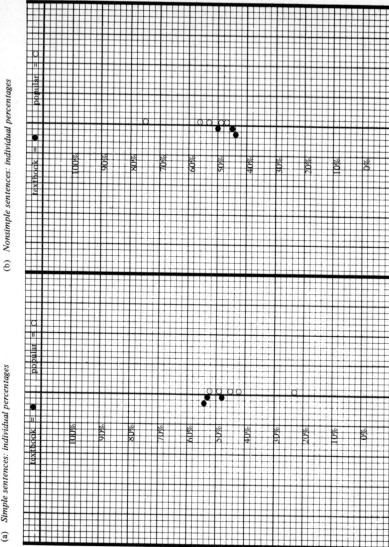

Table 4. (a) *Distribution in Disease Descriptions of sentences of pragmatic instruction: Imperious and nonimperious*

	T-1	T-2	T-3	Total	%[a]	P-1	P-2	P-3	P-4	P-5	Total	%[a]
Total no. of sentences in disease descriptions	667	660	855	2,182		274	29	125	313	51	792	
Sentences of pragmatic instruction	231	215	224	670	31	116	14	50	98	14	292	37
%[b]	35	33	26			42	48	40	31	27		

Table 4. (b) *Percentage of imperious vs nonimperious sentences*

	T-1	T-2	T-3	Total	%[a]	P-1	P-2	P-3	P-4	P-5	Total	%[a]
Total no. of sentences of pragmatic instruction	231	215	224	670		116	14	50	98	14	292	
Imperious sentences	92	64	102	258	39	51	4	32	43	9	139	48
%**	40	30	46			44	29	64	44	64		
Nonimperious sentences	139	151	122	412	61	65	10	18	55	5	153	52
%[b]	60	70	54			56	71	36	56	36		

[a] Based on group totals of numbers of sentences in Disease Descriptions.
[b] Based on individual totals of numbers of sentences in Disease Descriptions (see Table 2).

Graph 4.

(a) *Sentences of pragmatic instruction: individual percentages*

(b) *Imperious sentences: individual percentages*

(c) *Nonimperious sentences: individual percentages*

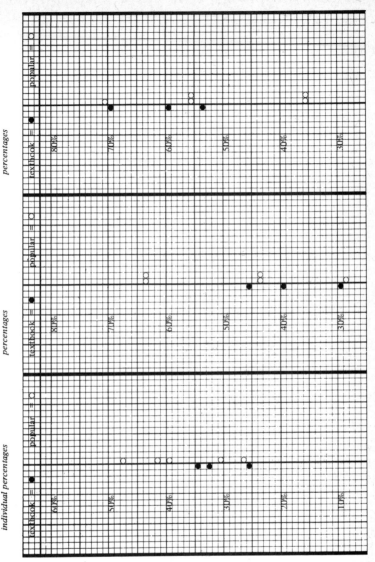

Table 5.   (a) *Distribution in Disease Descriptions of traditional sentence types: Assertive and nonassertive*

	T-1	T-2	T-3	Total	P-1	P-2	P-3	P-4	P-5	Total
Total no. of sentences	667	660	855	2,182	274	29	125	313	51	792
Assertive	661	659	852	2,172	253	29	119	291	51	743
Nonassertive	6	1	3	10	21	0	6	22	0	49
-Interrogative	0	1	0	1	4	0	6	4	0	14
-Imperative	6	0	3	9	17	0	0	15	0	32
-Exclamatory	0	0	0	0	0	0	0	3	0	3

Table 5. (b) *Percentage of assertive vs nonassertive sentences*

	T-1	T-2	T-3	Total	%[a]	P-1	P-2	P-3	P-4	P-5	Total	%[a]
Total no. of sentences in disease descriptions	667	660	855	2,182		274	29	125	313	51	792	
Assertive	661	659	852	2,172	99.5	253	29	119	291	51	743	93.8
%[b]	99.1	99.8	99.6			92.3	100	95.2	93	100		
Nonassertive	6	1	3	10	0.5	21	0	6	22	0	49	6.2
%[b]	0.9	0.2	0.4			7.7	0	4.8	7	0		

[a] Based on group totals of numbers of sentences in Disease Descriptions.
[b] Based on individual totals of numbers of sentences in Disease Descriptions (see Table 2).

Graph 5.
(a) *Assertive sentences: individual percentage*   (b) *Nonassertive sentences: individual percentages*

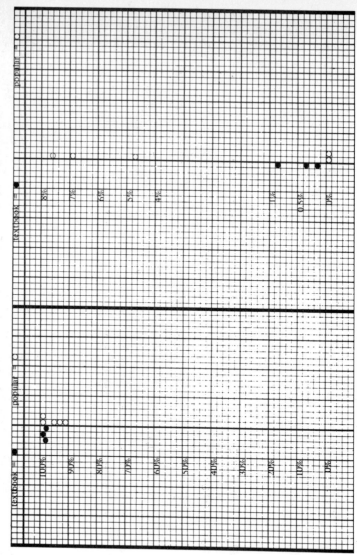

[iii] Terms belonging to the domain of exercise and physical activity. See Table 10.

[iv] The terms 'prevention', 'protection', 'health' or their variants. See Table 11.

[v] The term 'body'. See Table 12.

[vi] Terms referring to human subjects: Types A and B.[12] See Table 13.

[vii] Terms referring to human subjects: Types B_1 and B_2.[13] See Table 14.

The distribution in Disease Descriptions of lexical items which display the properties indicated above will now be demonstrated in Tables 6 to 14 and in their companion Graphs.

iii. *Other kinds of semiotic elements*

Thus far, Disease Descriptions of diabetes mellitus have been investigated according to the properties of their sentences and the properties of their lexical items. They will now be investigated according to a variety of other kinds of semiotic elements, namely:

[a] Quantifications expressed in Arabic numerals (see Table 15).

[b] Bracketed constructions, i.e. explanations, examples, or synonyms appearing in parentheses (see Table 16).

[c] Enumerated sets of words, phrases, etc. (see Table 17).

[d] Citations of works by other authors (see Table 18).

[e] The number of authors per Disease Description as compared to the total number of contributors per book (see Table 19).

The distribution in Disease Descriptions of the elements indicated above will now be demonstrated in Tables 15 to 19 and in their companion Graphs.

iv. *Properties of Schemata*

In order to determine which aspects of a Disease Description are typically emphasized by authors writing for textbooks of medicine, as compared to authors writing for popular home medical books, a cross-comparison was undertaken of the bold-type headings interspersed throughout each description of diabetes mellitus. As indicated earlier, each set of such headings has been designated by the term 'Schema' (plural 'Schemata'). (contd. on p. 77)

Table 6. *Distribution in Disease Descriptions of intersentential markers of coherence*

	T-1	T-2	T-3	Total	%[a]	P-1	P-2	P-3	P-4	P-5	Total	%[a]
	84	113	65	262	0.5	18	4	11	15	3	51	0.3
%[b]	0.6	0.6	0.3			0.4	0.7	0.4	0.2	0.3		

Table 7. *Distribution in Disease Descriptions of personal pronouns*

	T-1	T-2	T-3	Total	%[a]	P-1	P-2	P-3	P-4	P-5	Total	%[a]
	41	28	24	93	0.2	84	20	39	116	3	262	1.6
%[b]	0.3	0.1	0.1			2	3	1	2	3		

[a] Based on group totals of lexical items in Disease Descriptions.
[b] Based on individual totals of lexical items in Disease Descriptions (see Table 2).

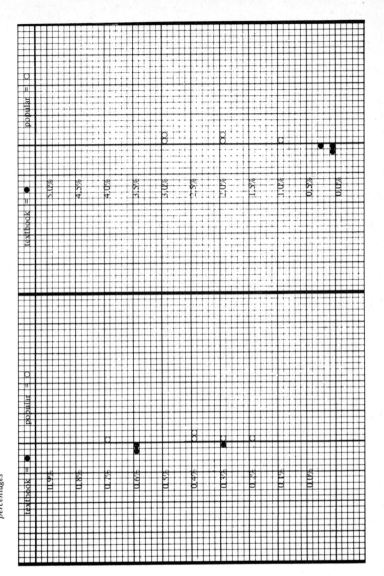

Graph 6. *Intersentential markers of coherence: individual percentages*

Graph 7. *Personal pronouns: individual percentages*

Table 8. *Distribution in Disease Descriptions of terms naming biochemicals*

	T-1	T-2	T-3	Total	%[a]	P-1	P-2	P-3	P-4	P-5	Total	%[a]
	684	761	953	2,398	4.5	182	31	69	127	19	428	2.6
%[b]	5	4	5			4	5	3	2	2		

Table 9. *Distribution in Disease Descriptions of terms belonging to the domain of food, food supplements, and dietetics*[c]

	T-1	T-2	T-3	Total	%[a]	P-1	P-2	P-3	P-4	P-5	Total	%[a]
	119	112	80	311	0.6	55	53	30	262	8	408	2.4
%[b]	1	1	0.4			1	9	1	3	1		

Table 10. *Distribution in Disease Descriptions of terms belonging to the domain of exercise and physical activity*

	T-1	T-2	T-3	Total	%[a]	P-1	P-2	P-3	P-4	P-5	Total	%[a]
	10	4	2	16	0.03	14	0	11	2	1	28	0.2
%[b]	0.1	0.02	0.01			0.3	0	0.4	0.03	0.1		

[a] Based on group totals of lexical items in Disease Descriptions.
[b] Based on individual totals of lexical items in Disease Descriptions (see Table 2).
[c] The terms 'carbohydrate', 'fat', and 'protein' have been included in Table 8 ('Terms naming biochemicals') rather than in Table 9.

Graph 8.　*Terms naming biochemicals: individual percentages*

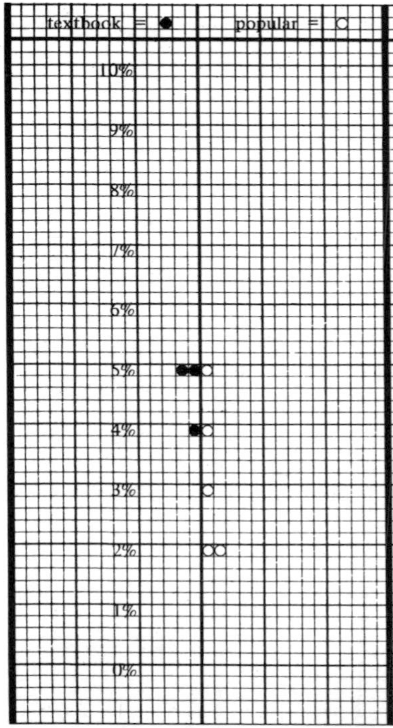

Graph 9.　*Terms belonging to the domain of food, food supplements, and dietetics: individual percentages*

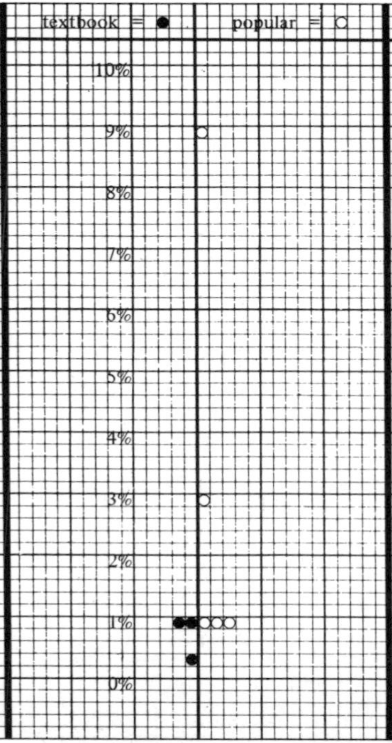

Graph 10.　*Terms belonging to the domain of exercise and physical activity: individual percentages*

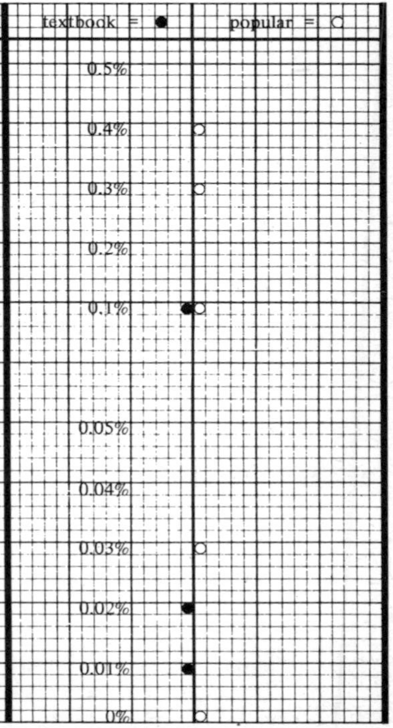

Table 11. *Distribution in Disease Descriptions of the terms 'prevention', 'protection', 'health' (and their variants)*

	T-1	T-2	T-3	Total	%[a]	P-1	P-2	P-3	P-4	P-5	Total	%[a]
	6	1	0	7	0.01	0	0	5	12	0	17	0.1
%[b]	0.04	0.01	0			0	0	0.2	0.2	0		

Table 12. *Distribution in Disease Descriptions of the term 'body'*

	T-1	T-2	T-3	Total	%[a]	P-1	P-2	P-3	P-4	P-5	Total	%[a]
	4	12	2	18	0.03	8	3	7	6	6	30	0.2
%[b]	0.03	0.1	0.01			0.2	0.5	0.3	0.1	0.7		

[a] Based on group totals of lexical items in Disease Descriptions.
[b] Based on individual totals of lexical items in Disease Descriptions (see Table 2).

Graph 11. *The terms 'prevention', 'protection', 'health' and their variants: individual percentages*

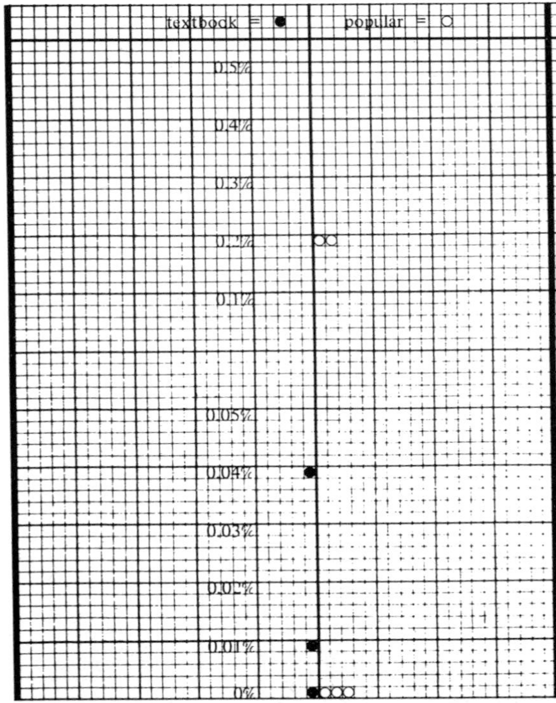

Graph 12. *The term 'body': individual percentages*

textbook = ●   popular = ○

0.7%   0.6%   0.5%   0.4%   0.3%   0.2%   0.1%   0.03%   0.02%   0.01%

textbook = ●   popular = ○

0.5%   0.4%   0.3%   0.2%   0.1%   0.05%   0.04%   0.03%   0.02%   0.01%   0%

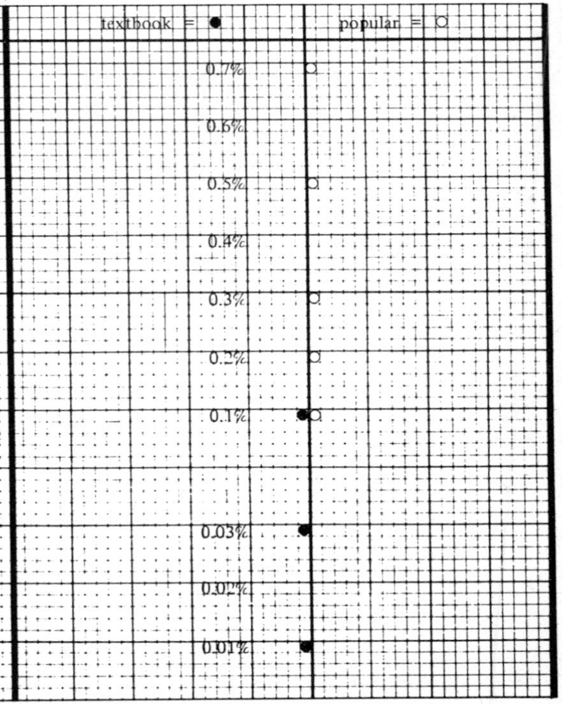

Table 13.   (a) *Distribution in Disease Descriptions of terms referring to human subjects: Type A and Type B*

	T-1	T-2	T-3	Total	$\%^a$	P-1	P-2	P-3	P-4	P-5	Total	$\%^a$
Total no. words in Disease Descriptions	14,938	18,762	19,768	53,468		4,940	604	2,759	7,528	888	16,719	
All terms referring to human subjects	239	281	256	776	1.5	138	10	113	35	30	326	1.9
$\%^b$	1.6	1.5	1.3			2.8	1.7	4.1	0.5	3.4		

Table 13.   (b) *Percentage of Type A vs Type B terms*

	T-1	T-2	T-3	Total	%[c]	P-1	P-2	P-3	P-4	P-5	Total	%[c]
All terms referring to human subjects	239	281	256	776	100	138	10	113	35	30	326	100
Type A terms	172	183	191	546	71	52	5	48	14	3	122	37
%[d]	72	65	75			38	50	42	40	10		
Type B terms	67	98	65	230	29	86	5	65	21	27	204	63
%[d]	28	35	25			62	50	58	60	90		

[a] Based on group totals of lexical items in Disease Descriptions.
[b] Based on individual totals of lexical items in Disease Descriptions.
[c] Based on group totals of terms referring to human subjects.
[d] Based on individual totals of terms referring to human subjects.

Graph 13.
(a) *Terms referring to human subjects:*
     individual percentages
(b) *Type A terms: individual percentages**
(b) *Type B terms: individual percentages**

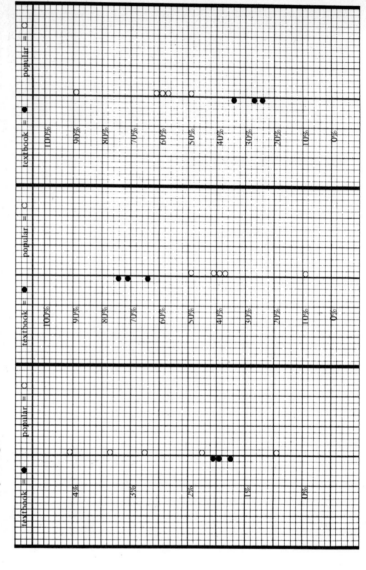

*Based on individual totals of terms referring to human subjects

Table 14. *Distribution in Disease Descriptions of terms referring to human subjects: Types B, B_1, and B_2*

	T-1	T-2	T-3	Total	%[a]	P-1	P-2	P-3	P-4	P-5	Total	%[a]
All Type B terms	67	98	65	230		86	5	65	21	27	204	
Type B_1 terms	41	66	50	157		41	4	59	20	11	135	
Type B_2 terms	12	1	6	19		13	1	4	0	16	34	
Total of B_1 and B_2 terms	53	67	56	176	23	54	5	63	20	27	169	83
%[b]	79	68	86			63	100	97	95	100		

[a] Based on group totals of Type B terms in Disease Descriptions.
[b] Based on individual totals of Type B terms in Disease Descriptions (see Table 13b).

Graph 14.   *Type (B$_1$ + B$_2$) terms: individual percentages**

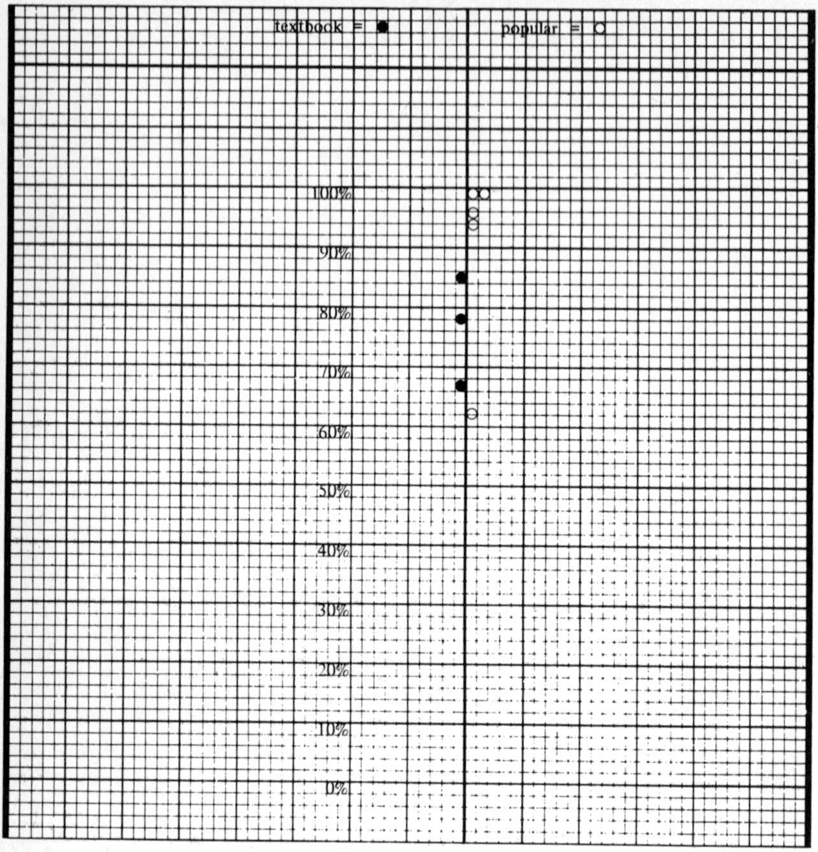

*Based on individual totals of Type B terms

Table 15. *Distribution in Disease Descriptions of quantifications expressed in Arabic numerals*[a]

	T-1	T-2	T-3	Total	%[a]	P-1	P-2	P-3	P-4	P-5	Total	%[b]
	335	146	223	704	1.3	21	1	1	35	3	61	0.4
%[c]	2	8	1			0.4	0.2	0.04	0.5	0.3		

Table 16. *Distribution in Disease Descriptions of bracketed constructions*[d]

	T-1	T-2	T-3	Total	%[b]	P-1	P-2	P-3	P-4	P-5	Total	%[b]
	73	53	71	197	0.4	1	0	3	20	0	24	0.1
%[c]	0.5	0.3	0.4			0.02	0	0.1	0.3	0		

[a] Quantifications expressed in natural language (e.g. 'fifty-five') have not been included in this Table.
[b] Based on group totals of lexical items in Disease Descriptions.
[c] Based on individual totals of lexical items in Disease Descriptions (see Table 2).
[d] Only those bracketed constructions containing either synonyms, explanations, or examples have been quantified. Excluded were bracketed references to books, pages, etc.

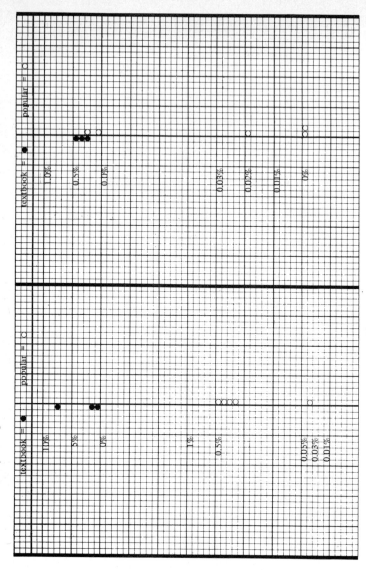

Graph 15.   *Quantifications expressed in Arabic numerals: individual percentages*

Graph 16.   *Bracketed constructions: individual percentages*

Table 17. *Distribution in Disease Descriptions of enumerated sets of words, phrases, etc.*

	T-1	T-2	T-3	Total	%[a]	P-1	P-2	P-3	P-4	P-5	Total	%[a]
	15	3	9	27	0.05	3	0	0	1	0	4	0.02
%[b]	0.1	0.01	0.05			0.06	0	0	0.01	0		

Table 18. *Distribution in Disease Descriptions of citations of works by other authors*[c]

	T-1	T-2	T-3	Total	%[a]	P-1	P-2	P-3	P-4	P-5	Total	%[a]
	14	16	63	93	0.2	0	0	0	22	0	22	0.1
%[b]	0.1	0.1	0.3			0	0	0	0.3	0		

[a] Based on group totals of lexical items in Disease Descriptions.
[b] Based on individual totals of lexical items in Disease Descriptions (see Table 2).
[c] In textbooks, citations of works by other authors follow the Disease Description; in P-4, they are all interspersed throughout the Disease Descriptions.

Graph 17.   Enumerated sets of words, phrases, etc.: individual percentages

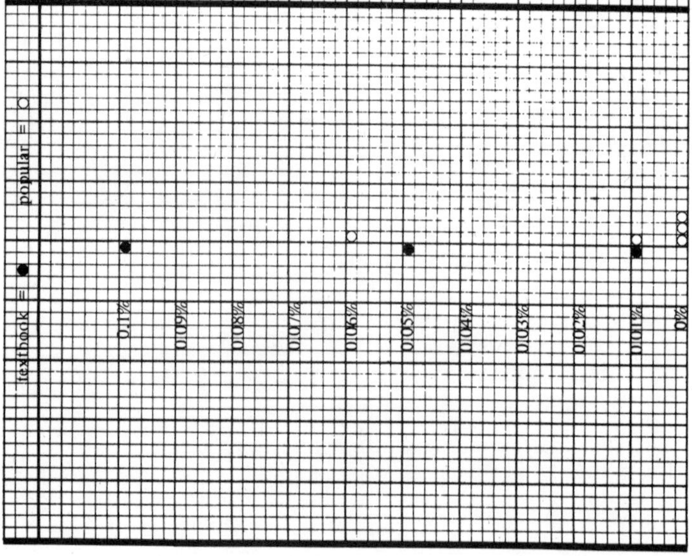

Graph 18.   Citations of works by other authors: individual percentages

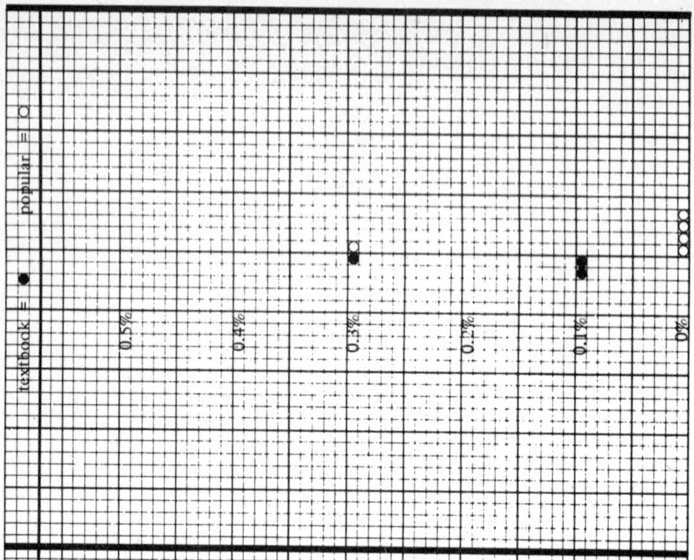

Table 19. *Number of authors per Disease Description as compared to total number of contributors per book*

	T-1	T-2	T-3	Total	Ave.	P-1	P-2	P-3	P-4	P-5	Total	Ave.
No. of authors per Disease Description	2	1	2	5	1.7	1	1	1	1	1	5	1
No. of authors per book	195	199	85	479	160	31	1	2	6	1	41	8
Ratio of no. of authors per Disease Description to no. of authors per book (in percentages)	1	0.5	2		1	3	100	50	17	100		54

Graph 19.
(a) *Number of authors per Disease
      Description*
(b) *Number of contributors per book*
(c) *Ratio of the number of authors/Disease
      Description: no. of contributors/book (%)*

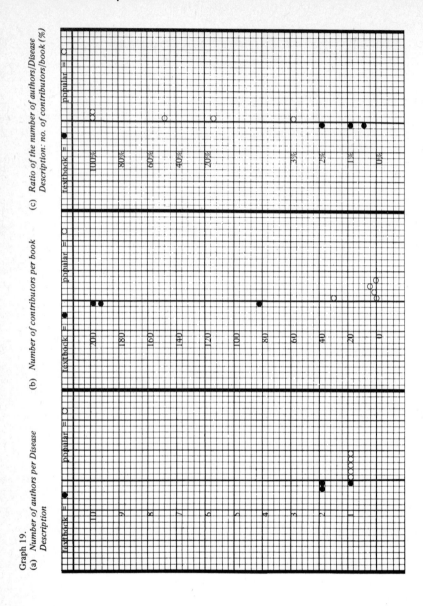

Owing to the diverse linguistic properties of the eight Schemata, it was necessary to recruit an 'external standard', one that would provide a common frame of reference, and thereby facilitate cross-comparison between the Schemata. The standard chosen was the set of chapter headings of a classical textbook on diabetes mellitus, *Joslin's Diabetes Mellitus,* and is reproduced in Table 20.

Table 20. *32 chapter headings of* Joslin's Diabetes Mellitus[a]

1. Current Concepts of Diabetes
2. Epidemiology and Detection of Diabetes
3. Pathophysiology of Diabetes Mellitus
4. Insulin in Diabetes—Applied Physiology
5. Glucagon
6. Glycoproteins and Diabetic Microangiopathy
7. The Pathology of Diabetes
8. Laboratory Procedures Useful in Diagnosis and Treatment
9. Onset, Course, Prognosis and Mortality in Diabetes Mellitus
10. General Plan of Treatment and Diet Regulation
11. Insulin in the Treatment of Diabetes
12. The Oral Hypoglycemic Agents
13. The Child with Diabetes
14. Diabetic Ketoacidosis and Coma
15. Cardiovascular Disease
16. The Eyes and Diabetes
17. Diabetic Nephropathy
18. The Nervous System and Diabetes
19. Pregnancy and Diabetes
20. Surgery and Diabetes
21. Infections and Diabetes
22. Disorders of the Blood
23. Disorders of the Skin in Diabetes
24. Diabetes and Other Endocrinologic Disorders
25. Cancer and Diabetes
26. Allergy and Diabetes
27. The Digestive System and Diabetes
28. Lipoatrophic Diabetes and Miscellaneous Conditions Related to Diabetes Mellitus
29. Emotional Factors in Diabetes Mellitus
30. Socioeconomic Considerations in the Life of the Diabetic
31. Hypoglycemia
32. Nondiabetic Melituria

contd.

Table 20 (*contd.*)

[a]Only Tables 2 through 19, 29, 39 through 56, and 58, 59 and 60 are accompanied by a companion Graph bearing the same number as the Table, and immediately following it. There are therefore no Graphs 20 through 28, 30 through 38, or 57.

All of the bold-type headings constituting the various Schemata[14] (reproduced respectively in Tables 21 to 28) have been enumerated by the writer in order to facilitate their being subsequently 'mapped'[15] (in Table 29) into the 32 chapter headings of *Joslin's*. Table 29 will make evident many differences (both in number and variety) concerning concepts which are emphasized in textbook as compared to popular Disease Descriptions. These differences will be interpreted further in Part Three, Section I: 1. It is important to note that while a concept may indeed be treated in a description without it necessarily being indicated by means of a bold-type heading, one intuitively assumes that those concepts which are so indicated reflect the author's intended emphasis.

Table 21.   *Schema of Disease Description of diabetes mellitus: T-1*

1.   History
2.   Prevalence
3.   Inheritance
4.   Classification
5.   Pathology
    (a)   Pancreas
    (b)   Blood vessels
        (i)   Retina
6.   Link Between Metabolic and Vascular Changes
7.   Pathophysiology
8.   Precipitation of Diabetes by Extrapancreatic Factors
    (a)   Obesity
    (b)   Pregnancy
9.   Diagnosis
10.   Fasting and postprandial blood glucose
    (a)   Oral glucose tolerance test
    (b)   Intravenous glucose tolerance test
11.   Differential diagnosis of glycosuria
12.   Clinical picture
    (a)   Juvenile-onset type
    (b)   Maturity-onset type

contd.

Table 21 (*contd.*)

13. Treatment
    (a) General principles
    (b) Diet
          Purpose
          Basic caloric requirement
          Partition of calories
          Carbohydrate
          Protein
          Fat
    (c) Oral hypoglycemic agents
          Sulfonylureas
          Tolbutamide
          Acetohexamide
          Chlorpropamide
          Tolazimide
    (d) Biguanides: Phenformin
    (e) Insulin
          Types of Insulin
          Choice of Insulin
          Initiation of insulin therapy
          Complications of insulin therapy
          (i) Insulin reactions
          (ii) Reactions at the site of insulin injection
          (iii) Insulin lipodystrophy
          (iv) Insulin resistance
14. Complications
    (a) Diabetic ketoacidosis and coma
          Diagnosis
          Differential diagnosis
          Treatment
    (b) Hyperglycemic hyperosmolar nonketotic coma
    (c) Lactic acidosis
    (d) Diabetic retinopathy
    (e) Diabetic nephropathy
    (f) Diabetic neuropathy
    (g) Gangrene of the feet
15. Surgery and diabetes mellitus
16. Pregnancy and diabetes mellitus
    (a) Diagnosis
    (b) Treatment

Table 22.   *Schema of Disease Description of diabetes mellitus: T-2*

---

1.   General Considerations
         History
2.   Pathophysiology
     (a)   Body Fuels
     (b)   Tissue fuel utilization
           (i)   Fed state
           (ii) Intravenous D and W
           (iii) Fasted state
     (c)   Diabetes
     (d)   Endocrine pancreas
           (i)   Insulin
           (ii) Glucagon
3.   Etiology
4.   Diagnosis
5.   Natural history and definitions
6.   Incidence and prevalence
7.   Clinical manifestations
     (a)   Eye
     (b)   Kidney
     (c)   Nervous system
     (d)   Skin
     (e)   Atherosclerosis
     (f)   Infection
8.   Lipoatrophic diabetes
9.   Secondary diabetes
     (a)   Hemochromatosis
     (b)   Pancreatitis
     (c)   Stress diabetes
     (d)   Acromegaly
     (e)   Cushing's syndrome
     (f)   Other endocrine and metabolic disorders
10. Treatment
     (a)   Diabetic ketoacidosis
     (b)   Hyperosmolar coma
     (c)   Nonketotic or nonhyperosmolar patient
     (d)   Oral hypoglycemic agents
11. Insulin Problems
     (a)   Allergy
     (b)   Insulin resistance
           (i)   Antibody-related
           (ii) Antibody-unrelated
           (iii) Obesity

contd.

Table 22 (*contd.*)

       (iv) Somogyi effect
  (c)   Lipoatrophy and hypertrophy
12. Hypoglycemia
13. Pregnancy and delivery
14. General principles in diabetic management

Table 23. *Schema of Disease Description of diabetes mellitus: T-3*

---

1. General Considerations and Classification
  (a)   Some aspects of intermediary metabolism
  (b)   Classification of diabetes mellitus
      (1)   Low-output failure
          (i)   Idiopathic islet cell failure
          (ii) Islet cell destruction
          (iii) Islet cell insufficiency
              (Failure to respond to stress)
          (iv) Islet cell insufficiency
              (Synthesis and release of impotent insulin)
          (v) The insensitive islet
              (Abnormal release of insulin from the pancreas)
          (vi) The blocked islet
      (2)   High-output failure
          (i)   The association of obesity with diabetes mellitus
          (ii) High-output failure in association with known insulin antagonists
          (iii) The role of glucagon in diabetes mellitus
          (iv) Lipodystrophies associated with diabetes
      (3)   Hypertriglyceridemia in diabetes
2. Clinical presentation of diabetes mellitus
3. The diagnosis of diabetes mellitus
  (a)   Fasting plasma glucose
  (b)   Glucose tolerance test
  (c)   The steroid provocative tests
4. Treatment of diabetes mellitus
  (a)   Dietary regimens in diabetes mellitus
          (i)   The overweight diabetic
          (ii) The underweight diabetic
  (b)   The oral hypoglycemic agents
          (i)   Tolbutamide
          (ii) Chlorpromadine
          (iii) Acetohexamide

contd.

Table 23 (*contd.*)

               (iv) Tolazamide
               (v) Phenformin

  (c)   The use of insulin in diabetes mellitus
  (d)   Problems of insulin therapy
               (i)   Insulin hypoglycemia
               (ii) Unusual degrees of insulin resistance
               (iii) Insulin hives
               (iv) Local fat changes at sites of injection

5. Diabetic comas
     Diabetic ketoacidosis
               (i)   Treatment of diabetic acidosis
               (ii) The glucose hyperosmality syndrome
               (iii) Diabetic lactic acidosis

6. Late manifestations of diabetes mellitus
  (a)   Coronary artery disease
  (b)   Peripheral vascular disease
  (c)   Renal disease
  (d)   Eye disease
  (e)   Neurological disease
               (i)   Mononeuritis Multiplex
               (ii) Amyotrophy
               (iii) Predominant autonomic neuropathy
  (f)   Other situations facing the diabetic
               (i)   Pregnancy
               (ii) Surgery

Table 24.   *Schema of Disease Description of diabetes mellitus: P-1*

---

1. Diabetes
  (a)   Diagnosis
  (b)   Symptoms
2. Management of the Diabetic Patient
  (a)   Diagnosis
  (b)   Exercise
  (c)   Insulin types
  (d)   Insulin
  (e)   Individualization of doses
  (f)   Oral hypoglycemic agents
  (g)   Selection of oral agents
  (h)   Urine tests
  (i)   Complications

contd.

Table 24 (*contd.*)

   (j)   Diabetic coma
   (k)   Insulin reactions
   (l)   Blood vessel complications
   (m)   Care of the feet
   (n)   Infections

Table 25.   *Schema of Disease Description of diabetes mellitus: P-2*

1.   How to Use Diet to Relieve Fatigue Caused by Diabetes
2.   The medicinal value of green vegetables
3.   Balancing diet and insulin
4.   How to boost a diabetic diet's efficiency with food supplements

Table 26.   *Schema of Disease Description of diabetes mellitus: P-3*

1.   Diabetes in Later Life
2.   Pregnancy
3.   Foot Care
4.   Tertiary Prevention

Table 27.   *Schema of Disease Description of diabetes mellitus: P-4*

1.   A Deadly Disease You Can Live With
   (a)   Insatiable thirst is an early symptom
   (b)   Diabetes can strike at any age
2.   What is a diabetic diet? Delicious!
   (a)   Delicious as well as healthful
   (b)   Weight control is crucial
   (c)   Not all carbohydrates are bad
   (d)   Eat more raw foods
3.   Brewer's yeast has what it takes to normalize blood sugar
   (a)   Insulin can't function without chromium
   (b)   Chromium brought 'overnight recovery'
   (c)   Deficiency is widespred in U.S.
4.   Vitamin E for arterial disease in diabetics
   (a)   Treatment is incomplete without vitamin E
   (b)   Visual deterioration halted
5.   Diabetics, here's how to save your feet
   (a)   Gangrene may develop

contd.

Table 27 (*contd.*)

    (b)   Feet need daily care
    (c)   Vitamin C speeds wound healing
    (d)   Vitamin E can save limbs

Table 28.   *Schema of Disease Description of diabetes mellitus: P-5*

1.   The Pancrease—Diabetes
2.   Symptoms of Diabetes
3.   Excessive Insulin

Table 29.   *Mapping procedure between Schemata* and Joslin's headings*

Joslin's 32 chapter headings	T-1	T-2	T-3	P-1	P-2	P-3	P-4	P-5
1. Current Concepts of Diabetes	1 4	1	1	1				
2. Epidemiology and Detection of Diabetes	2 3 8	3 6	3				1b	
3. Pathophysiology of Diabetes Mellitus	7	2a 2b 2c	1a 1b					
4. Insulin in Diabetes— Applied Physiology								
5. Glucagon		2d (ii)	1b (2) (iv)					
6. Glycoproteins and Diabetic Microangiography								
7. The Pathology of Diabetes	5a							1

contd.

*Note that all numbers appearing in this Table refer to the enumerated bold-type headings of each Schema (see Tables 21 to 28).

Table 29 (*contd.*)

Joslin's 32 chapter headings	T-1	T-2	T-3	P-1	P-2	P-3	P-4	P-5
8. Laboratory Procedures Useful in Diagnosis and Treatment	9 10	4	3	1a 2h				
9. Onset, Course, Prognosis and Mortality in Diabetes Mellitus	12	5	2	1b			1a	2
10. General Plan of Treatment and of Diet Regulation	12a 13b	10c 14	4a	2a 2b 2m	1 2 4	3	2 3 4a	
11. Insulin in the Treatment of Diabetes	13e	11	4c 4d	2c 2d 2e	3			3
12. The Oral Hypoglycemic Agents	13c 13d	10d	4b	2f 2g				
13. The Child with Diabetes								
14. Diabetic Ketoacidosis and Coma	14a 14b 14c	10a 10b	5	2j 2k				
15. Cardiovascular Disease	5b 6	7e	6a 6b	2l				
16. The Eyes and Diabetes	5b(i) 14d	7a	6d				4b	
17. Diabetic Nephropathy	5c 14e	7b	6c					
18. The Nervous System and Diabetes	14f	7c	6e					
19. Pregnancy and Diabetes	16	13	6f(i)			2		

contd.

Table 29 (*contd.*)

Joslin's 32 chapter headings	T-1	T-2	T-3	P-1	P-2	P-3	P-4	P-5
20. Surgery and Diabetes	14g 15		6f (ii)				5	
21. Infection and Diabetes		7f		2n				
22. Disorders of the Blood								
23. Disorders of the Skin in Diabetes		7d						
24. Diabetes and Other Endocrinological Disorders		9c 9d 9e 9f						
25. Cancer and Diabetes								
26. Allergy and Diabetes		11a	4d (iii)					
27. The Digestive System and Diabetes		9a 9b						
28. Lipoatrophic Diabetes and Miscellaneous Conditions Relating to Diabetes Dellitus		8	1b (2) (v)					
29. Emotional Factors in Diabetes Mellitus								
30. Socioeconomic Considerations in the Life of the Diabetic								
31. Hypoglycemia		12	4d (i)					

contd.

Table 29 (*contd.*)

Joslin's 32 chapter headings	T-1	T-2	T-3	P-1	P-2	P-3	P-4	P-5
32. Nondiabetic Melituria	11							
Total number of *Joslin's* headings which are 'covered' by the Schema of each Disease Description	17	22	19	8	2	3	5	3
Percentage	53	69	59	15	6	9	16	9

To summarize:

A semiotic comparison of the Texts in all eight selected books was effected by means of cross-comparing a representative portion from each of the Texts (namely, each Disease Description of diabetes mellitus), one with another.

Four kinds of comparisons were subsequently undertaken:

i. according to properties of sentences;
ii. according to properties of lexical items;
iii. according to other kinds of semiotic elements;
iv. according to properties of Schemata.

All data accruing from these comparisons have been presented in Tables 2 to 29, in their companion Graphs, and in Supplement A. This data will be interpreted in Part Three as constituting evidence pointing towards differences in form and contents in textbooks as compared to popular books.

Having investigated the semiotic properties of the Texts, the writer will turn next to a comparison of the semiotic properties of the Tables of Contents, p. 98.

SUPPLEMENT A

A-1
Disease Descriptions: Sample Paragraphs

(a) Textbooks

T-1   'The aims in managing diabetes are (1) to correct the underlying meta-

Graph 29.   *Percentage of Joslin's chapter headings which are 'covered' by each Schema of diabetes mellitus*

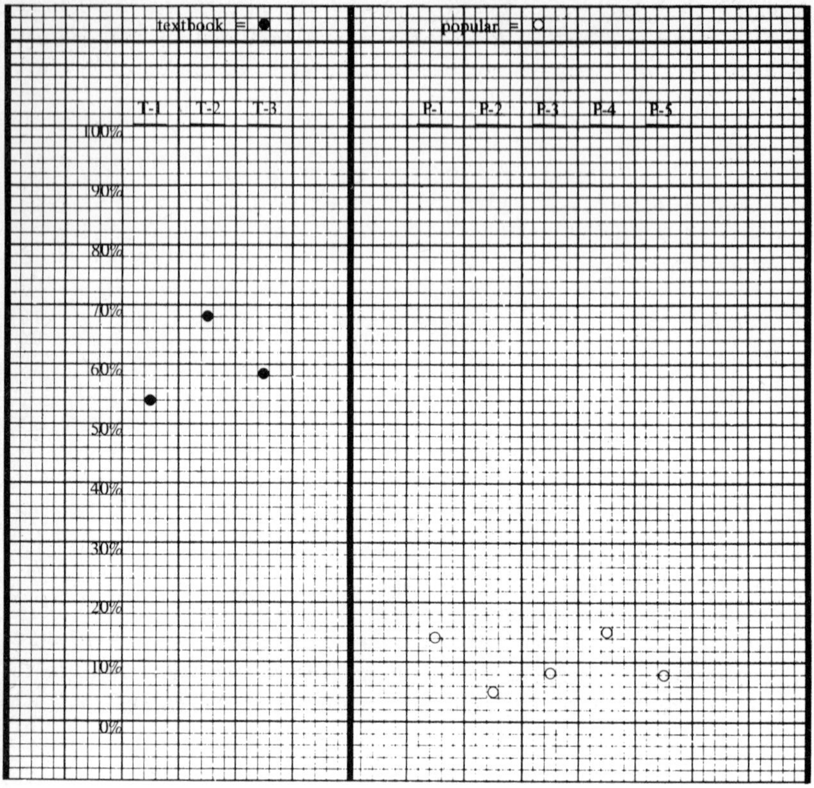

bolic abnormalities in order to reduce diabetic symptoms; (2) to attain and maintain ideal body weight; (3) to prevent, or at least delay, specific complications commonly associated with the disease (disorders of eye, kidney, nerves); and (4) to stem the nonspecific accelerated atherosclerosis to which the diabetic is particularly liable'.

T-2 'In the terminal ketoacidotic patient in coma, the thready pulse, decreasing blood pressure, rapidly falling arterial pH, and rising PCO_2 (signifying inability to achieve compensation of the acidosis by hyperventilation) portend irreversible shock and death, and rapid heroic treatment is mandatory to reverse the fatal outcome. On the other hand, many patients will walk in with mild ketoacidosis, feeling poorly, without nausea or vomiting, but with a glucose level of 500 mg per 100 ml or higher and a total HCO_3 of 4 to 16 mEq per liter . . .'

T-3 'The physician should appraise the clinical picture every 30 minutes. Table 9 provides a useful guideline for intravenous therapy. Insulin is given at hourly intervals until the plasma acetoacetate falls to 3 mmoles per liter or less or until the urine ketone is reduced. Some of the metabolic changes that occur with insulin deprivation are reversed only after several hours of insulin therapy. Thus the continuing presence of circulating insulin may be more important than the actual level. A recent report demonstrating effective management of ketoacidosis with an initial intramuscular dose of 10 to 20 Units and 5 to 10 Units every hour thereafter supports this concept'.

(b) *Popular books*

P-1 'Diabetes mellitus is an inherited disease which occurs when the body cannot make full use of some of the foods we eat—mainly the carbohydrates or sugars and starches. The pancreas, a large gland lying beneath the stomach, does not make available enough insulin to burn these foods as energy or store them for future use. Starches and sugars increase the blood sugar content until the sugar passes through the kidneys and into the urine. This loss of carbohydrate energy causes the symptoms of diabetes and can lead to an illness which can be fatal if it is not properly controlled'.

P-2 'When the pancreas is constantly abused or overworked from excessive use of sugar, it eventually becomes exhausted and fails to produced enough insulin to cope with large amounts of sugar. Then, what began as low blood sugar from an overproduction of insulin becomes diabetes or *high* blood sugar from a deficiency of insulin. In either case, you'll have to *avoid sugar and refined carbohydrates* and go easy on natural starches in order to keep your blood sugar under control. With the average American consuming about 150 pounds of sugar annually, it's no wonder hypoglycemia and diabetes are so common. Hypoglycemia is rarely detected and treated by physicians, but diabetes is often detected in routine medical examinations'.

P-3   'In diabetes, something is wrong with the body's ability to use (or meta- bolize) sugar. In a typical, overt case of diabetes, the level of sugar in the blood will be too high and sugar (glucose) will "spill over" from the blood into the urine. On the other hand, in many cases of diabetes, the defect in sugar utilization will become apparent only with a glucose tolerance test. In this test, blood sugar is first determined after several hours of fasting and then again at intervals after the patient is given three and one-half ounces of glucose solution to drink. By studying the curve drawn between the measure- ments at various times, the doctor can detect a diabetic tendency. If the test is positive and the patient as yet has no symptoms of diabetes, he is said to have preclinical or chemical diabetes'.

P-4   'In the simplest terms, diabetes results when the body is unable to make full use of the carbohydrates (sugars and starches) we eat. Either because the pancreas does not produce enough insulin to process these sugars for storage or use in the cells, or because the insulin produced is less effective than it should be, the sugar (glucose) stays in the blood, accumulating there until it spills over into the kidneys and the urine. The body cannot afford this con- tinued loss of valuable carbohydrates and eventually diabetes symptoms are likely to occur'.

P-5   'Studies of diabetes show that heredity plays an important part. The relationship is becoming more and more clear as people with diabetes tend to live longer and have more children. Once diabetes in childhood was considered invariably fatal. Now these children grow up, marry, and have families. We now know that if both parents are diabetic, the children will most certainly inherit the disease. Overweight is also important in relationship to diabetes. Not everyone who is overweight develops the disease. In fact, diabetes is seen in only a small proportion of the people who are overweight. However, nine out of ten people who develop diabetes are overweight. Among those who are overweight and who develop diabetes, dieting and restoration to normal weight lessens the severity of the symptoms and sometimes controls the con- dition. The person who is overweight, however, can produce more and more insulin and this may be a factor in exhausting the function of the pancreas.

As I have mentioned in previous articles, both the pituitary gland and the adrenal glands are also related in their functions to the use of sugar by the body. Excessive action of the pituitary gland may result in the appearance of sugar in the urine. Excessive action of the thyroid gland may make diabetes worse by increasing the work of the gland, through the fact that the person is taking in large amounts of food'.

A-2

Disease Descriptions: Sentences of Pragmatic Instruction—Imperious vs Nonimperious Types

Sentences of pragmatic instruction represent a fairly large proportion of all sentences found in Disease Descriptions.[16] Such sentences are clearly intended to influence the reader in carrying out certain practical actions, that is, they are intended to provoke pragmatic consequences.[17] These sentences have been investigated according to the 'manner' in which the instructional message is transmitted. Hence, the following two types: imperious and nonimperious.

Sentences of the imperious type typically afford the reader no option in the carrying out of the instruction. They include both imperative as well as normative sentences. In the former (frequently called 'commands'), the subject, 'you', is characteristically omitted, as in: 'Test the patient's urine four times daily'; 'Never wear ill-fitting shoes'.

Normative sentences are of two kinds: (a) those which contain the verbal forms 'should', 'must', 'need', 'require', 'demand', 'necessitate', or a form of the infinitive 'to have', as in the following: 'Insulin *should* (*must, has to*) be given at this time'; 'The patient *need not* fast'; 'Such cases *require* (*demand, necessitate*) prompt action'; and (b) those which contain a subject, the copula 'is', and any of the following complements: 'necessary', 'imperative', 'demanded', 'essential', 'mandatory', 'obligatory', 'required', 'crucial', or 'vital', as in: 'It is *necessary* (*imperative, etc.) that a normal blood sugar be maintained'. Another variety of complement includes either of the infinitives 'to be' or 'to have', followed by the past participle of certain transitive verbs, as in 'Blood *is to be drawn* before breakfast'; 'The patient *has to be told*'.

Sentences of the nonimperious type, as their name suggests, are considerably less emphatic, less verbally coercive, than those of the imperious type. They include two subtypes: advisory and exemplary.

Sentences of the advisory type afford the reader at least some option in carrying out the instruction, as is evident by the softer degree of emphasis. Examples include: 'It is *wise* (*helpful, desirable, sensible, important, reasonable*) to recommend a specialist in these cases'; 'Prompt ingestion of glucose is *recommended* (*effective, advised, suggested, indicated, useful, beneficial, of benefit, advisable,* etc.) during such occurrences'; '*It's a good idea* to have your eyes checked at regular intervals'; '*One of the worst things to do* is to drink alcohol'; 'The diabetic *would do well* to keep his weight down'; 'You *may* (*can*) begin immediately'; 'In such cases, an increase in the daily dosage is *warranted* (*justified, defensible, indicated*)'; 'Orange juice is *allowed* (*permitted*)'.

Sentences of the exemplary type are typically 'neutral' with respect to emphasis, yet are nevertheless clearly intended for pragmatic instruction. Examples include the following: 'Glucose (0.5 g per kg in 3 min) *is infused* and blood samples for glucose determination *are drawn* at frequent intervals for 2 to 3 hours'; 'The diabetes *is treated* according to its signs and symptoms, until the primary cause of the excess glucocorticoid is corrected'; 'A drop of urine *is placed* on the tablet and within one minute a purple color appears if there is acetone in the urine'; 'Immediate attention *is given* to all bruises and cuts of the skin'. These kinds of sentences have been called 'exemplary' because they all express prototypical messages concerning what is (ideally or customarily) done in certain situations.

These sentence types appear to correspond to three traditional methods of teaching: (a) by imposing imperatives (sentences of imperious type); (b) by suggestion (sentences of the advisory type); and (c) by example (sentences of the exemplary type).

A-3
Disease Descriptions: Sentences Manifesting a Colloquial Style[18]

P-1

1. 'Properly treated, diabetics can expect to live *just about as long* as anyone else.'
2. 'That is *the direct opposite* of diabetes.'
3. 'Insulin reactions are *just the opposite* of diabetic coma.'
4. '*It may lead to trouble* in various parts of the body.'
5. 'Socks that are too small or too large *may cause trouble*.'

P-2

1. '*How to* Use Diet to Relieve Fatigue Caused by Diabetes.'
2. '. . . *you'll* have to . . . *go easy on* natural starches . . .'
3. '. . . *it's no wonder* hypoglycemia and diabetes are so common.'
4. 'You can test for urine sugar *right in your own home* . . .'
5. 'Natural food supplements can be used to . . . *boost the healing powers* of the body.'

6. '*How to boost* a diabetic diet's efficiency with food supplements.'

7. '*It's* important that . . . they *stay away from* refined sugar . . .'

8. 'Such foods *won't flood your blood* with sugar.'

P-3

1. 'Physicians know *all too well* the unpleasant outlook for the patient . . .'

2. '. . . *it's a good idea* to avoid crowded places.'

3. '*There is worry that* one or more of these oral medicines may not be as helpful as insulin.'

4. '. . . *the way to a long life* is to get a chronic disease and *learn to live with it.*'

5. 'Some "diabetics" have even been able *to quit* taking insulin.'

P-4

1. A *Deadly Disease* You Can *Live* With.'

2. '. . . modern scientific advances have made diabetes a disease that *can be lived with,* and *doors are opening* to the ultimate control of the problem . . .'

3. 'Insurance companies are generally *willing to bet* that diabetics who follow their doctor's advice *will live to a ripe old age.*'

4. '*What is a Diabetic Diet? Delicious.*'

5. 'The chances that you will ever have to *walk the metabolic tightrope* of this chronic disease are less than one in fifty.'

6. 'But if diabetes should *strike, you would be doing yourself a favor* by following your doctor's dietary advice . . .'

7. '. . . a diabetic diet—conscientiously followed—*can be a real life pre-server.*'

8. '. . . a diabetic who makes an extra effort to take care of himself *is really a step ahead . . . on the road to health.*'

9. 'First, *let's clear up once and for all* the widely-held notion that a diabetic diet has to be unappealing.'

10. 'In the book . . . Euell Gibbons *tells the story of his brother Joe . . .*'

11. 'Gibbons was *in for a surprise!*'

12. 'My love of good food was *beginning to show around my middle.*'

13. 'Dinner was *a revelation!*'

14. 'The overweight diabetic who successfully *peels off enough pounds* . . . usually experiences a dramatic improvement. . .'

15. 'Too concentrated a source of sugar will quickly . . . *send the blood glucose skyrocketing out of control.*'

16. '*It's true that* starch . . . end(s) up as glucose.'

17.   '. . . the next highest rating was for black pepper, *of all things!*'

18.   '*But* does chromium have the same anti-diabetic effect in humans? Yes, there is firm evidence establishing this fact.'

19.   '. . . all . . . had (*among their other woes*) faulty glucose metabolism.'

20.   'Brewer's Yeast *Has What It Takes* to Normalize Blood Sugar.'

21.   '*Chromium Brought "Overnight Recovery".*'

22.   '*It goes without saying* that chromium will be effective . . .'

23.   '*But* brewer's yeast is *far and away* the best source of . . .'

24.   '*But*, like all hormones, this one *can't do its job* alone.'

25.   'Arteriosclerosis has become the *major killer of diabetics* . . .'

26.   'In an attempt to give diabetes a *better-than-even* chance of surviving the heart problems . . . some medical authorities are *taking a second look at* Vitamin E . . .'

27.   'One disease is . . . treated by diet and insulin and *all that sort of thing.*'

28.   '. . . degeneration of the blood vessels . . . *is what kills.*'

29.   'This is what *knocks out* the eyes and the kidneys and the heart . . .'

30.   '*No diabetic is being treated at all* unless he takes alpha tocopherol.'

31.   '. . . and he was feeling *really well.*'

32.   'In no way, however, can the suggestion be made to *do away with* insulin. *It's* needed.'

33.   'The millions of persons the hormone has helped *cannot be anything but thankful* . . .'

34.   '*But it still makes good sense* to try to *combat* . . . heart and artery disease.'

35.   '*Diabetics, Here's How to Save Your Feet.*'

36.   'To someone with a painful corn on his foot, his freedom from pain may seem *a blessing,* but to the diabetic, it is *a menace.*'

37.   '. . . when the warning signal of pain is also *out of kilter,* the danger is very real.'

38.   '. . . the flow of blood to the feet (is) *choked off by clogged arteries.*'

39.   'If you have diabetes and smoke, *you might as well tie rubber bands around your ankles* . . .'

40.   'One researcher who has no doubt that ascorbic acid *will go a long way* toward *putting some spunk into the limp resistance* of the diabetic is . . .'

P-5

1.   'As *I* have mentioned in previous articles . . .'

A-4

Disease Descriptions: Sentences Which Impart Reassurance, Encouragement, and Hope to the Reader[19]

P-1

1. 'There are heartening aspects, however. First, most diabetics no longer die of their diabetes, but of some ailment or complication common to other people. Second, most authorities believe that the closer a diabetic follows the rules laid down by his doctor, the more likely he is to postpone or avoid complications.'

2. 'Early diagnosis, prompt and proper treatment have prolonged the life of the diabetic considerably. Properly treated, diabetics can expect to live just about as long as anyone else and as usefully and happily . . .'

3. 'Diet is still the basis of treatment of diabetes. Insulin is needed in some individuals, but in a large proportion of patients, particularly older ones, the diabetes can be controlled by a diet and an oral drug. Successful treatment depends not only on diet, insulin, and drugs, but also on the favorable outlook of the individual patient.'

4. 'Diabetics do best when they put aside concern for their condition, trust in the doctor with whom they are cooperating, and lead normally active lives. Virtually every calling in life is open to them.'

P-2

1. 'Some "diabetics" are even able to quit taking insulin when they change their eating habits.'

2. 'Natural food supplements can be used to overcome nutritional deficiencies and to boost the healing powers of the body.'

P-3

1. 'Tertiary Prevention: Perhaps someday it will become possible to transplant a normal pancreas to the diabetic who suffers from deficient secretion of insulin. As a surgical feat, pancreas transplantation presents no great problems. It is the body's tendency to reject the transplant that is the big problem—here as with other transplants—that must be solved.'

2. 'All that we have written and admonished may seem so forbidding that a diabetic may ask, 'Is life worth living?' We can assure him that it is. Many people with diabetes have distinguished themselves in sports, in industry, in the arts. They accept their disease—and the extra discipline needed to live successfully with it. As one wise physician has observed, the way to a long life is to get a chronic disease and learn to live with it.'

P-4

1. 'A Deadly Disease You Can Live With.'

2. 'Diabetes is unwelcome at any age, but modern scientific advances have made diabetes a disease that can be lived with, and doors are opening to the ultimate control of the problem in all its phases. A diabetic willing to watch his diet and take the minimal precautions that any health-conscious individual would take anyway, can live virtually a normal life with virtually a normal life expectancy.'

3. 'Perhaps the most encouraging, most convincing evidence of that outlook comes from the insurance companies. Diabetes patients are usually insurable. Insurance companies are generally willing to bet that diabetics who follow their doctors' advice will live to a ripe old age.'

4. 'What is a Diabetic Diet? Delicious!'

5. 'Most people never get diabetes. The chances that you will ever have to walk the tightrope of this chronic disease are less than one in fifty.'

6. 'A number of new research findings and recommendations by physicians indicate that a diabetic diet—conscientiously followed—can be a real life preserver. In fact, the diabetic who makes an extra effort to take care of himself is really a step ahead of his nondiabetic counterpart on the road to health. It's not surprising that a diabetic diet should be so beneficial. It has to be.'

7. 'The overweight diabetic who successfully peels off enough pounds to get his weight back to normal usually experiences a dramatic improvement in his condition. Indeed, the symptoms often virtually disappear.'

A-5

Disease Descriptions: Sentences Which Reinforce to the Reader the Role of the Doctor

P-1

1. 'The best way to find out if you have diabetes is to report to your doctor or clinic and have him do the urine and blood test examination.'

2. 'However, be careful to consult your doctor.'

3. 'The answer to the individual's problems in this regard must be worked out with the aid of a doctor.'

4. 'When such increased demands are noted, unless the reason is obvious—for example a cold or mild respiratory infection—the patient must consult his doctor.'

5. 'Since so many factors are involved in individual insulin requirements, it is wise to leave the regulation of its amount in the hands of a skilled physician.'

6.   'Thus, when you are ill, do not attempt to regulate the insulin dose by checking only your personal feelings or urine tests—consult your physician.'

7.   'Your physician is the only guide to this problem.'

8.   'Second, most authorities believe that the closer a diabetic follows the rules laid down by his doctor, the more likely he is to postpone or avoid complications.'

9.   'Call a doctor immediately to be certain other procedures are not necessary.'

10.   'Never put strong medications such as iodine or carbolic acid on your feet without first consulting your doctor.'

11.   'If a high fever is present, if the infection persists over a period of two or three days, and large quantities of urine are passed, a physician should be notified.'

12.   'Proper treatment calls for a close working relationship between the diabetic patient and his physician.'

P-2

1.   'These people should be under the care of a physician so that blood sugar measurements can be used to determine the amount of insulin they need.'

2.   'An occasional blood sugar examination by your doctor will help you evaluate your eating habits.'

P-3

1.   'The patient must have complete confidence in the physician, since few diseases require more close cooperation between patient and doctor.'

2.   'Since there are several types of insulin—fast-acting, slow-acting, and intermediate—the doctor can determine which one or which combination is best suited for the individual patient.'

3.   'The patient should learn from the doctor exactly how to measure insulin into a syringe, the type to purchase, how and where to give the injection, and how to vary the injection site so that no one area of skin is used too much.'

4.   'Every diabetic on oral medication should review the situation with his doctor; a consultation with a specialist in diabetes may be recommended and should be accepted by the patient.'

5.   'The key to prevention of many complications during pregnancy lies in close cooperation between obstetrician and other physician and the pregnant woman.'

6. 'It is another reason why a prospective diabetic mother should notify her doctor the moment she suspects she may be pregnant.'

7. 'Ideally, the diabetic patient should go regularly to a foot specialist, a podiatrist, for preventive care of the feet.'

8. 'If an infection develops, there should be no delay in seeing a doctor or podiatrist.'

9. 'Unfortunately, there are additional difficulties which some diabetics may experience, and which they should recognize and discuss promptly with the doctor.'

10. 'He should feel no shame in mentioning this to his doctor; if necessary, he should discuss the problem with a psychotherapist.'

11. 'Swelling of the ankles may be an indication of a kidney complication of diabetes, called Kimmelstiel-Wilson syndrome, and should be reported promptly to the doctor.'

P-4

1. 'Once a diagnosis of diabetes has been made, the doctor and the patient join in a mutual effort to restore a carbohydrate balance to the system, all the while maintaining a good nutritional status.'

2. 'Insurance companies are generally willing to bet that diabetics who follow their doctors' advice will live to a ripe old age.'

3. 'But if diabetes should strike, you would be doing yourself a great favor by following your doctor's dietary advice precisely.'

4. 'If that's the case, he must get someone else to do the job, or see a podiatrist regularly.'

5. 'Visit a podiatrist.'

P-5

1. 'The physician should be asked to make all of the necessary studies to determine the severity of the condition and to prescribe treatment promptly in order to control the disease.'

2. 'Patients must co-operate with the doctor in regulating the control of sugar in relation to insulin intake.'

2.   THE TABLE OF CONTENTS

a.   *Its purpose*

The purpose of the set of headings which constitutes each Table of Contents is to indicate the topical scope and organization of the Text. For example, the inclusion of the major heading 'Immune Disease' in the Table of Contents of T-1, and of the major heading 'Infections and Immunity' in the Table of Contents of P-5, indicates that each of these books includes medical statements addressed to a special subdomain or topic of the semantic domain of Medicine, namely, 'immunology'.[20] However, the Table of Contents of P-5 also happens to contain the major heading 'Your Vacation', which is unique to that particular book. Hence, P-5 differs from the other books of medical instruction in that its scope includes a topic (which we might call 'the medical significance of a vacation') which is not addressed in any of the other books. Therefore, each Table of Contents of the eight selected books not only addresses a different scope but, in addition, organizes that scope according to different classificatory principles.[21]

b. *Its composition*

The Tables of Contents of all eight selected books are comprised of various major headings, subheadings, and, especially in the case of textbooks, of numerous sub-subheadings. These headings, in turn, are composed either of individual lexical items, of phrases, or of clauses. Only the major or first level headings will be investigated in this section.[22]

c. *Selected Headings: Rationale for investigation*

All headings to be investigated (hereafter called Selected Headings) will be analyzed with three objectives in mind: (i) to determine how textbooks differ from popular books with respect to their broad scope, i.e. with respect to the combination of major topics in terms of which the Text has been constructed; (ii) to determine how textbooks and popular books differ with respect to the linguistic properties of the main lexical items which constitute their Selected Headings;[23] and (iii) to identify, amongst the main lexical items in the Selected Headings, three taxonomic classes: Class T (exclusive to Selected Headings of textbooks, Class P (exclusive to Selected Headings of popular books, and class $T \cap P$ (common to Selected Headings of both).

i. *Objective no. one: A comparison of scope*
Owing to the diversity of linguistic properties in the Selected Headings of all books, it was found necessary, once again,[24] to recruit an 'external standard', such that in providing a common frame of reference, it would facilitate cross-comparison between the various sets of Selected Headings. The standard

selected for this purpose was the 'List of Three-digit Categories', a set of 17 headings used in the international statistical classification of disease. This standard is reproduced in Table 30 below.

Table 30.   *17 headings of the 'List of Three-digit Categories'*[25]

I.	Infectious and Parasitic Disease
II.	Neoplasms
III.	Endocrine, Nutritional and Metabolic Diseases, and Immunity Disorders
IV.	Diseases of the Blood and Blood-Forming Organs
V.	Mental Disorders
VI.	Diseases of the Nervous System and Sense Organs
VII.	Diseases of the Circulatory System
VIII.	Diseases of the Respiratory System
IX.	Diseases of the Digestive System
X.	Diseases of the Genitourinary System
XI.	Complications of Pregnancy, Childbirth, and the Puerperium
XII.	Diseases of the Skin and Subcutaneous Tissue
XIII.	Diseases of the Musculoskeletal System and Connective Tissue
XIV.	Congenital Anomalies
XV.	Certain Conditions Originating in the Perinatal Period
XVI.	Symptoms, Signs and Ill-defined Conditions
XVII.	Injury and Poisoning

Tables 31 to 38 contain, respectively, the Selected Headings of each of the eight books of medical instruction.

A detailed mapping procedure[26] has been undertaken between each of these eight sets of Selected Headings and the set of 17 'Categories' of the 'List of Three-digit Categories', and appears in Supplement B-1. Table 39 provides an abbreviated form of this mapping procedure, further elaborated in Graphs 39(a) and (b) respectively.

This mapping procedure has enabled the writer not only to explore the differences in scope between textbooks and popular books in a systematic way, but also to express these differences vis-à-vis that set of standardized expressions for topics which the 'List' provides. Differences discovered with respect to the scope of textbooks as compared to popular books will be interpreted in Part Three, Section II: 1.

Table 31. *T-1: Table of Contents: Selected Headings**

* In mapping the headings of the Table of Contents of T-1 on to the 17 'Categories' of the 'List', a decision was made to include the *sub*headings of Parts Three and Seven in order to demonstrate more adequately the correlations between the Table of Contents of T-1 and the 'List'.

Table 32. *T-2: Table of Contents: Selected Headings*[†]

contd.

Table 32 (*contd.*)

Part	VIII.	*Microbial Diseases*
Part	IX.	*Protozoan and Helminthic Diseases*
Part	X.	*Disorders of the Nervous System and Behavior*
Part	XI.	*Respiratory Disease*
Part	XII.	*Cardiovascular Diseases*
Part	XIII.	*Renal Diseases*
Part	XIV.	*Diseases of the Digestive System*
Part	XV.	*Diseases of Nutrition*
Part	XVI.	*Hematologic and Hematopoietic Diseases*
Part	XVII.	*Diseases of Metabolism*
Part	XVIII.	*Diseases of the Endocrine System*
Part	XIX.	*Diseases of Bone*
Part	XX.	*Certain Cutaneous Diseases with Significant Systemic Manifestations*
Part	XXI.	*Miscellaneous Hereditary Disorders Affecting Multiple Organ Systems*
Part	XXII.	*Normal Laboratory Values of Clinical Importance*

[†] No subheadings were required in the mapping of the Table of Contents of T-2 on to the 17 'Categories' of the 'List'.

Table 33. *T-3: Table of Contents: Selected Headings* [‡]

Section One:	*The Approach to the Patient*
Section Two:	*Disorders of Water and Electrolyte Metabolism*
Section Three:	*Renal Diseases and Disturbances in Renal Function*
Section Four:	*Cardiovascular Disease*
Section Five:	*Pulmonary Disease*
Section Six:	*Medical Genetics*
Section Seven:	*Hematology*
Section Eight:	*Neoplastic Diseases*
Section Nine:	*Diseases of the Gastrointestinal Tract*
Section Ten:	*Diseases of the Liver*
Section Eleven:	*Endocrinology*
Section Twelve:	*Infectious Diseases*
Section Thirteen:	*Diseases with Abnormalities of Immunity*
Section Fourteen:	*Rheumatic Disease*
Section Fifteen:	*Disorders of the Nervous System*
Section Sixteen:	*Psychiatry in Medicine*
Section Seventeen:	*Diseases of Medical Management*
Section Eighteen:	*Medical Emergencies*
Section Nineteen:	*Special Topics in Medicine*

contd.

Table 33 (*contd.*)

‡ In mapping the headings of the Table of Contents of T-3 on to the 17 'Categories' of the 'List', a decision was made to include the *sub*headings of Section Nineteen in order to demonstrate more adequately the correlations between the Table of Contents of T-3 and the 'List'.

Table 34.   *P-1: Table of Contents: Selected Headings* *

* No subheadings were required in the mapping of the Table of Contents of P-1 on to the 17 'Categories' of the 'List'.

Table 35.   *P-2: Table of Contents: Selected Headings*†

---

† No subheadings were required in the mapping of the Table of Contents of P-2 on to the 17 'Categories' of the 'List'.

Table 36.   *P-3: Table of Contents: Selected Headings*‡

---

contd.

Table 36 (*contd.*)

contd.

Table 36 (*contd.*)

10. Bone Diseases
11. Breast Diseases
12. Chronic Bronchitis and Emphysema
13. Brucellosis (Undulant Fever)
14. Bursitis
15. Cancer
16. Cerebral Palsy
17. Clubfoot and Congenital Hip Dislocation
18. Common Cold
19. Cushing's Syndrome (Adrenal Cortical Hyperfunction)
20. Diabetes
21. Dizziness and Meniere's Disease
22. Epilepsy
23. Gallbladder Disease
24. Gonorrhea and Other Venereal Diseases
25. Headache (Including Migraine)
26. Heart Diseases
27. Hemophilia and Related Diseases
28. Hemorrhoids
29. Hernia
30. High Blood Pressure (Hypertension)
31. Hodgkin's Disease
32. Kidney Disease
33. Leprosy (Hansen's Disease)
34. Leukemia
35. Liver Disease
36. Low Blood Pressure
37. Malaria
38. Menopause
39. Menstrual Disorders and Fibroids
40. Infectious Mononucleosis
41. Motion Sickness
42. Multiple Sclerosis
43. Muscle Disorders
44. Myasthenia Gravis
45. Narcolepsy (and Related Conditions)
46. Parkinson's Disease
47. The Pneumonias
48. Poliomyelitis
49. Prostate Gland Enlargement
50. Psoriasis
51. Purpura

contd.

Table 36 (*contd.*)

‡ In mapping the headings of the Table of Contents of P-3 on to the 17 'Categories' of the 'List', a decision was made to include the *sub*headings of Parts 2, 3, 4, and 5 in order to demonstrate more adequately the correlations between the Table of Contents of P-3 and the 'List'.

* Part One, which contains Chapters 1 through 5, will be treated as a preface or introduction, since the book contains no *formal* Preface or Introduction. Thus, the statements in Part One of P-3 will be treated in Part Two: 3 of this study with respect to establishing the *editorial stance* of the book.

† The following items have been provided with numbers in order to facilitate mapping.

Table 37.   *P-4: Table of Contents: Selected Headings*‡‡

contd.

Table 37 (*contd.*)

32.	Goiter	48.	Parkinson's Disease
33.	Hair and Scalp Problems	49.	Prostate Disorders
		50.	Rabies
34.	Hay Fever	51.	Sexual Disorders
35.	Headache	52.	Shingles
36.	The Heart	53.	Sinusitis
37.	Hemorrhoids	54.	The Skin
38.	Hernia	55.	Avoiding Ailments of Teeth and Gums
39.	Hospital-Caused (Nosocomial) Infections	56.	Tetany
40.	Insomnia	57.	Tonsillitis
41.	Kidney Disease	58.	Toxemia of Pregnancy
42.	The Liver	59.	Tuberculosis
43.	Miscarriage	60.	Ulcers
44.	Mononucleosis	61.	Varicose Veins
45.	Motion Sickness	62.	Venereal Diseases
46.	Multiple Sclerosis	63.	Weight Problems
47.	Muscular Dystrophy		

‡‡ No subheadings were required in the mapping of the Table of Contents of P-4 on to the 17 'Categories' of the 'List'.

Table 38.   *P-5: Table of Contents: Selected Headings**

contd.

Table 38 (*contd.*)

* No subheadings were required in the mapping of the Table of Contents of P-5 on to the 17 'Categories' of the 'List'.

Table 39. *Mapping Procedure Between Selected Headings and the 'List of Three-Digit Categories'*

17 'Categories' of the 'List'	Selected Headings							
	T-1	T-2	T-3	P-1	P-2	P-3	P-4	P-5
I. Infectious and Parasitic Diseases	●	●	●	●	○	●	●	●
II. Neoplasms	●	○	●	●	○	●	●	●
III. Endocrine, Nutritional and Metabolic Diseases, and Immunity Disorders	●	●	●	●	●	●	●	●
IV. Diseases of the Blood and Blood-forming Organs	●	●	●	●	○	●	●	○
V. Mental Disorders	●	●	●	●	●	●	●	●
VI. Diseases of the Nervous System and Sense Organs	●	●	●	●	○	●	●	●
VII. Diseases of the Circulatory System	●	●	●	●	●	●	●	●

contd.

Graph 39.

(a) *Percentage of 'Three-digit Categories' which are 'covered' by the Selected Headings of each book*

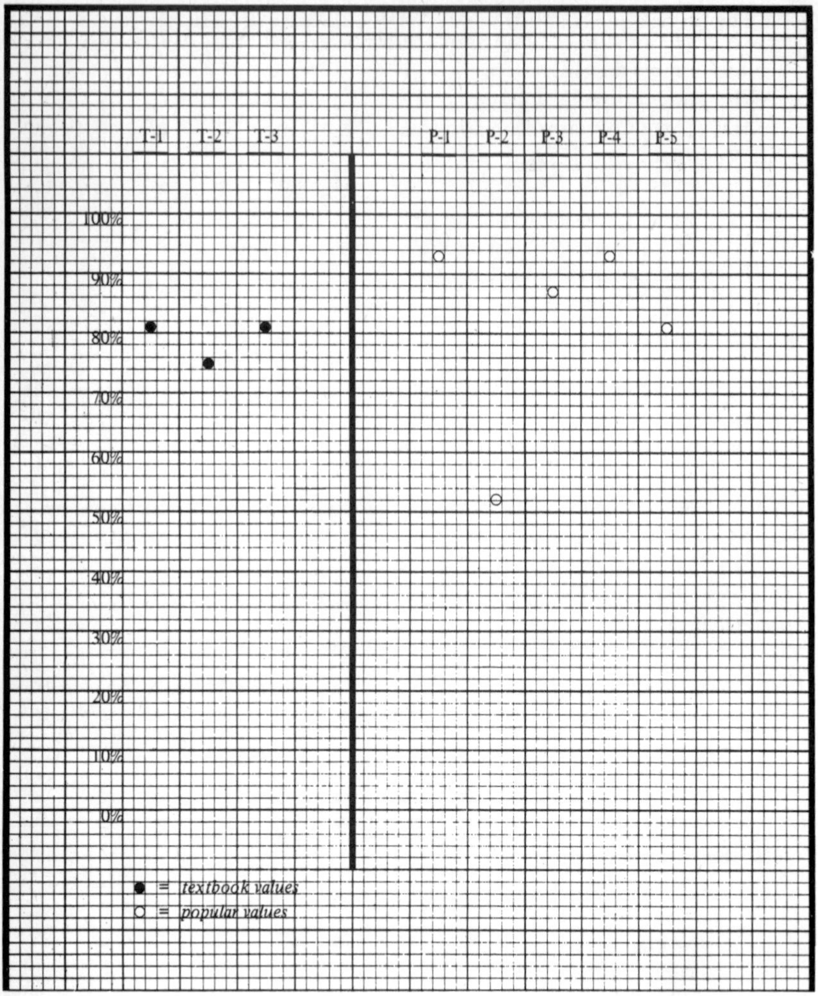

Table 39 (*contd.*)

17 'Categories' of the 'List'	Selected Headings							
	T-1	T-2	T-3	P-1	P-2	P-3	P-4	P-5
VIII. Diseases of the Respiratory System	●	●	●	●	●	●	●	●
IX. Diseases of the Digestive System	●	●	●	●	●	●	●	●
X. Diseases of the Genitourinary System	●	●	●	●	○	●	●	●
XI. Complications of Pregnancy, Childbirth, and the Puerperium	○	○	○	●	○	○	●	○
XII. Diseases of the Skin and Subcutaneous Tissue	○	●	●	●	●	●	●	●
XIII. Diseases of the Musculoskeletal System and Connective Tissue	●	●	●	●	●	●	●	●
XIV. Congenital Anomalies	●	●	●	●	○	●	●	●
XV. Certain Conditions Originating in the Perinatal Period	○	○	○	●	○	○	○	○
XVI. Symptoms, Signs and Ill-defined Conditions	●	○	○	○	●	●	●	●
XVII. Injury and Poisoning	●	●	●	●	●	●	●	●
Percentage of 'Three-digit Categories' which are 'covered' by the Selected Headings of each book	82	76	82	94	53	88	94	82

● = the book in question contains a Selected Heading which corresponds to the 'Category'.

○ = the book in question contains *no* Selected Headings which correspond to the 'Category'.

ii. *Objective no. two: A comparison of linguistic properties*
Selected Headings of textbooks of medicine and popular home medical books will now be compared in terms of the linguistic properties of their constituent lexical items. *Method:* All terms (whether individual lexical items or sequences of lexical items) bearing the linguistic properties which are indicated below have been counted in each of the eight sets of Selected Headings.

Graph 39.
(b) *Percentage of representation of each 'category' in Selected Headings: textbook vs popular*

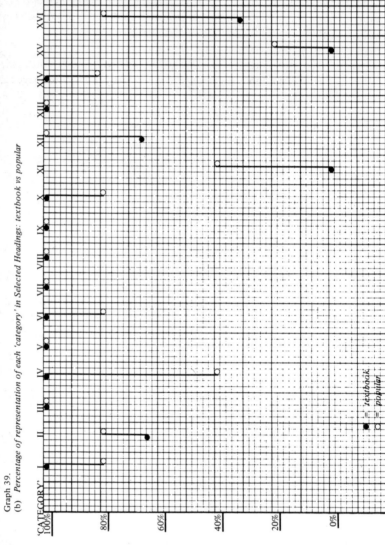

Group percentages have been based on the number of main lexical items in Selected Headings of all three textbooks, on the one hand, and of all five popular books, on the other. Individual percentages have been based upon the number of main lexical items in each of the eight individual sets of Selected Headings. See Table 40 for the results of these basic calculations.

With respect to each identified linguistic property, all data are presented in three complementary formats: [a] a Table, [b] a Graph, and [c] a Supplement. The data in each Table are presented numerically, but are displayed in a more visually communicative manner in a companion Graph which follows that Table and bears the same number as the Table. Supplements have been provided for many of the Tables in order to exemplify the property which has been calculated.

Below, then, are listed the various linguistic properties of Selected Headings which have been investigated, indicating the particular Tables or Supplements in which data pertaining to that property are to be found.

Linguistic properties of Selected Headings have been compared in terms of the following features: [a] phonological, [b] grammatical, and [c] semantic.

[a]   Analyses of *phonological* properties have been restricted to a measurement of the distribution of monosyllabic words (see Supplement B-4 and Table 41).

[b]   Analyses of *grammatical* properties involve a measurement of the distribution of terms belonging to the following grammatical categories:

   [i]   personal pronouns (see Supplement B-5 and Table 42).

   [ii]   gerunds (see Supplement B-6 and Table 43).

   [iii]   compound nouns (see Supplement B-7 and Table 44).

   [iv]   prepositional phrases (see Supplement B-8 and Table 45).

   [v]   adverbial clauses containing an infinitive (see Supplement B-9 and Table 46).

[c]   Analyses of *semantic* properties involve a measurement of the distribution of terms belonging to the following semantic classes:

   [i]   Terms which name aberrant states, or which name indicators of aberrant states, Type One (see Supplement B-10 and Table 47).

   [ii]   Terms which name aberrant states, or which name indicators of aberrant states, Type Two (see Supplement B-11 and Table 48).

   [iii]   Terms belonging to the domain of treatment or care of the human organism (see Supplement B-12 and Table 49).

   [iv]   The terms 'health', 'prevention', or their variants (see Supplement B-13 and Table 50).

   [v]   The term 'body' (see Supplement B-14 and Table 51).

   [vi]   The term 'system' and its variants (see Supplement B-15 and Table 52).

[vii] Nouns which name anatomical structures of the human organism: 'covert' vs 'overt' structures (see Supplement B-16 and Table 53).

[viii] Terms which belong to the domains of psychiatry, neurology, and behavioral psychology (see Supplement B-17 and Table 54).

[ix] Terms which name certain sexual, social, and developmental states or roles of the human organism (see Supplement B-18 and Table 55).

[x] Terms which name so-called 'natural' approaches to the maintenance of health (see Supplement B-19 and Table 56).

All data contained in the above Tables, in the companion Graphs, and in their indicated Supplements will be interpreted in Part Three to show how textbooks differ from popular books both in form as well as in contents.

Table 40. *Numbers of main lexical items in Selected Headings: Individual and group totals*

T-1	T-2	T-3	Total	P-1	P-2	P-3	P-4	P-5	Total
82	70	56	208	71	142	232	93	84	622

Table 41. *Distribution in Selected Headings of monosyllabic words*

	T-1	T-2	T-3	Total	%*	P-1	P-2	P-3	P-4	P-5	Total	%*
	8	2	1	11	5	30	56	44	19	26	175	28
%†	10	3	2			42	39	24	20	31		

* Based on group totals of main lexical items in Selected Headings.
† Based on individual totals of main lexical items in Selected Headings (see Table 40).

Table 42. *Distribution in Selected Headings of personal pronouns*

	T-1	T-2	T-3	Total	%ᵃ	P-1	P-2	P-3	P-4	P-5	Total	%‡
	0	0	0	0	0	7	4	4	0	3	18	3
%**	0	0	0			10	3	2	0	4		

‡ Based on group totals of main lexical items in Selected Headings.
** Based on individual totals of main lexical items in Selected Headings (see Table 40).

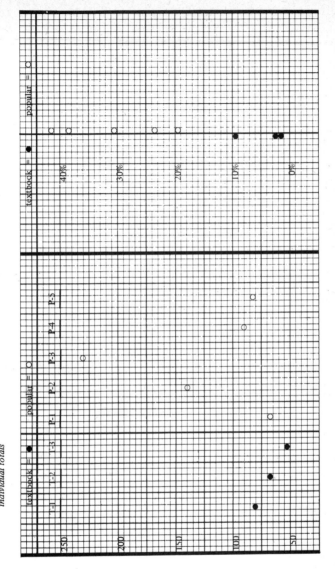

Graph 40. *Numbers of main lexical items in Selected Headings: individual totals*

Graph 41. *Monosyllabic words: individual percentages*

Table 43.   *Distribution in Selected Headings of gerunds*

	T-1	T-2	T-3	Total	%*	P-1	P-2	P-3	P-4	P-5	Total	%*
	0	0	0	0	0	0	12	5	4	4	25	4
%†	0	0	0			0	8	2	4	5		

Table 44.   *Distribution in Selected Headings of compound nouns*

	T-1	T-2	T-3	Total	%*	P-1	P-2	P-3	P-4	P-5	Total	%*
	4	4	2	10	5	4	14	23	14	6	61	10
%†	5	6	4			6	10	10	15	7		

Table 45.   *Distribution in Selected Headings of prepositional phrases*

	T-1	T-2	T-3	Total	%*	P-1	P-2	P-3	P-4	P-5	Total	%*
	16	12	11	39	19	4	22	0	2	11	39	6
%†	20	17	20			6	15	0	2	13		

Table 46.   *Distribution in Selected Headings of adverbial clauses containing an infinitive*

	T-1	T-2	T-3	Total	%*	P-1	P-2	P-3	P-4	P-5	Total	%*
	0	0	0	0	0	0	11	0	0	0	11	2
%†	0	0	0			0	8	0	0	0		

* Based on group totals of main lexical items in Selected Headings.
† Based on individual totals of main lexical items in Selected Headings (see Table 40).

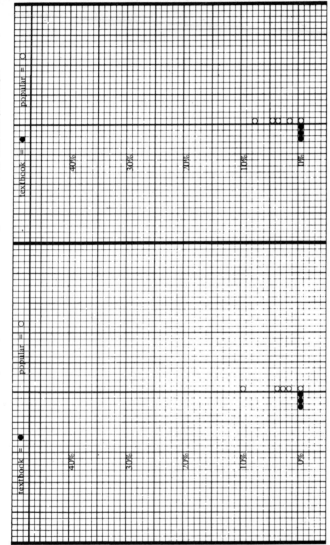

Graph 42. *Personal pronouns: individual percentages*

Graph 43. *Gerunds: individual percentages*

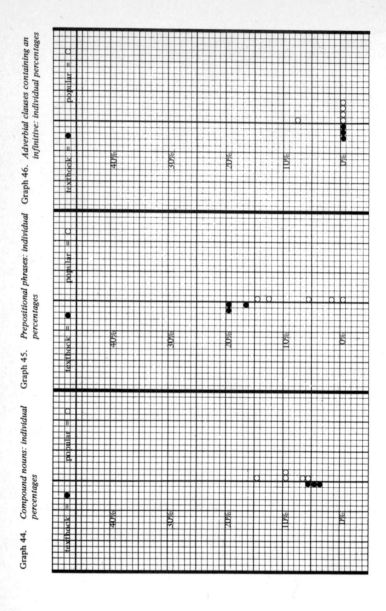

Graph 44. *Compound nouns: individual*   Graph 45. *Prepositional phrases: individual*   Graph 46. *Adverbial clauses containing an*
percentages   *percentages*   *infinitive: individual percentages*

Table 47. *Distribution in Selected Headings of Type One terms which name aberrant states, or which name indicators of aberrant states: 'Standard' vs 'nonstandard' terms*

	T-1	T-2	T-3	Total	%[a]	P-1	P-2	P-3	P-4	P-5	Total	%[a]
Total no. of Type One terms	21	21	16	58	28	6	14	25	16	15	76	12
%[b]	26	30	29			8	10	11	17	18		
'Standard' Type One terms	21	21	14	56		5	5	18	10	12	50	
%[c]	100	100	88			83	36	72	63	80		
'Nonstandard' Type One terms	0	0	2	2		1	9	7	6	3	26	
%[c]	0	0	12			17	64	28	37	20		

[a] Based on group totals of main lexical items in Selected Headings.
[b] Based on individual totals of main lexical items in Selected Headings (see Table 40).
[c] Based on individual totals of Type One terms in Selected Headings.

Graph 47.   TYPE ONE TERMS FOR ABERRANT STATES OR FOR INDICATORS OF ABERRANT STATES
(a)   *Type One terms: individual percentages*   (b)   *'Standard' Type One terms: individual*   (c)   *'Nonstandard' Type One terms: individual*
*percentages**   *percentages**

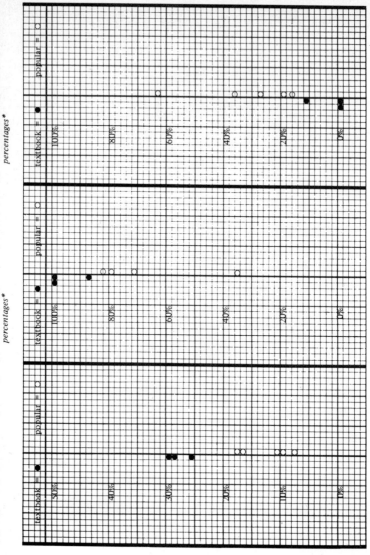

*Based on individual totals of Type One terms

Table 48. *Distribution in Selected Headings of Type Two terms which name aberrant states, or which name indicators of aberrant states*

	T-1	T-2	T-3	Total	%[a]	P-1	P-2	P-3	P-4	P-5	Total	%[a]
	0	1	0	1	1	5	16	65	41	5	132	21
%[b]	0	1	0			7	11	28	44	6		

Table 49. *Distribution in Selected Headings of terms belonging to the domain of treatment or care of the human organism*

	T-1	T-2	T-3	Total	%[a]	P-1	P-2	P-3	P-4	P-5	Total	%[a]
	1	0	1	2	1	6	27	9	0	2	44	7
%[b]	1	0	2			8	19	4	0	2		

Table 50. *Distribution in Selected Headings of the terms 'Health', 'Prevention', or their variants*

	T-1	T-2	T-3	Total	%[a]	P-1	P-2	P-3	P-4	P-5	Total	%[a]
	0	0	0	0	0	1	0	12	1	1	15	2
%[b]	0	0	0			1	0	5	1	1		

Table 51. *Distribution in Selected Headings of the term 'Body'*

	T-1	T-2	T-3	Total	%[a]	P-1	P-2	P-3	P-4	P-5	Total	%[a]
	0	0	0	0	0	0	1	4	0	3	8	1
%[b]	0	0	0			0	1	2	0	4		

[a] Based on group totals of main lexical items in Selected Headings.
[b] Based on individual totals of main lexical items in Selected Headings (see Table 40).

Graph 48.   *Type Two terms: individual percentages*

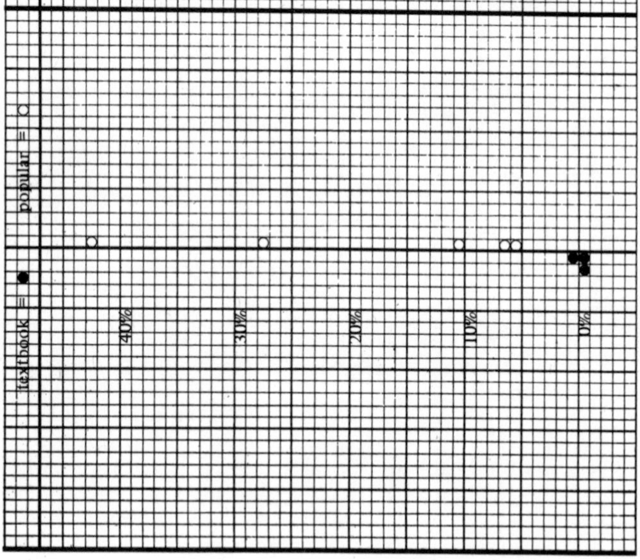

Graph 49.   *Terms belonging to the domain of treatment or care of the human organism: individual percentages*

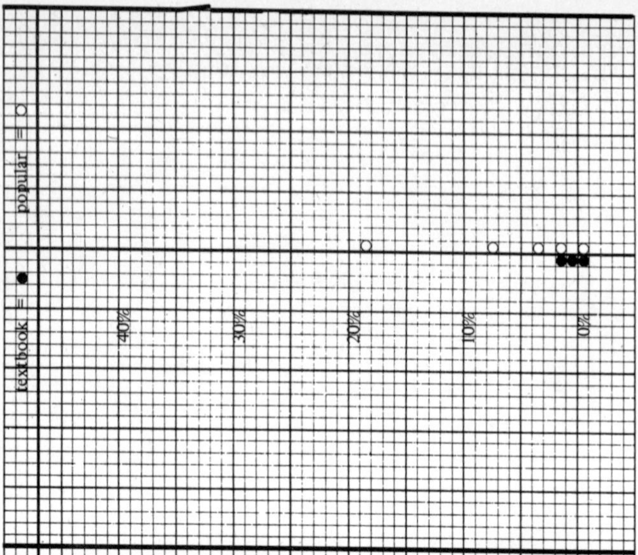

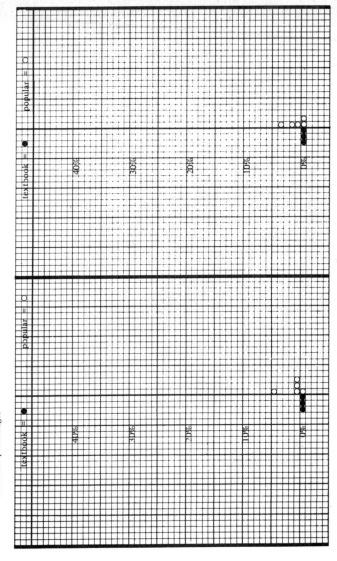

Graph 50.   The terms 'health', 'prevention' and their variants: individual percentages

Graph 51.   The term 'body': individual percentages

Table 52.   (a) Distribution in Selected Headings of the term 'System' (or variant)

	T-1	T-2	T-3	Total	%[a]	P-1	P-2	P-3	P-4	P-5	Total	%[a]
The term 'System' (or variant)	6	5	1	12	6	3	0	6	1	0	10	2
%[b]	7	7	2			4	0	3	1	0		

Table 52.   (b) Terms indicating kinds of systems: 'Standard' vs 'nonstandard' terms

	T-1	T-2	T-3	Total	%[a]	P-1	P-2	P-3	P-4	P-5	Total	%[a]
'Standard' terms indicating kinds of systems	2	2	1	5		3	0	5	1	0	9	
%[c]	33	50	100			100	0	83	100	0		
'Nonstandard' terms indicating kinds of systems	4	2	0	6		0	0	1	0	0	1	
%[c]	67	50	0			0	0	17	0	0		

[a] Based on group totals of main lexical items in Selected Headings.
[b] Based on individual totals of main lexical items in Selected Headings (see Table 40).
[c] Based on individual totals of terms indicating kinds of systems.

Graph 52.

(a) *The term 'System': individual percentages*

(b) *'Standard' terms naming kinds of systems: individual percentages**

(c) *'Nonstandard' terms naming kinds of systems: individual percentages**

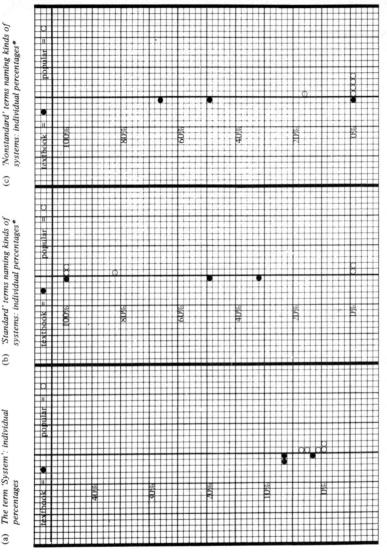

*Based on individual totals of terms naming kinds of systems

Table 53. *Distribution in Selected Headings of nouns which name anatomical structures of the human organism: 'Covert' vs 'overt' structures*

	T-1	T-2	T-3	Total	%[a]	P-1	P-2	P-3	P-4	P-5	Total	%[a]
Total no. of nouns naming anatomical structures	10	3	3	16	8	15	15	24	15	11	80	13
%[b]	12	4	5			21	11	10	16	13		
Nouns naming 'covert' structures	10	3	2	15	93[d]	8	6	15	7	5	41	51[d]
%[c]	100	100	67			53	40	63	47	45		
Nouns naming 'overt' structures	0	0	1	1	7[d]	7	9	9	8	6	39	49[d]
%[c]	0	0	33			47	69	37	53	55		

[a] Based on group totals of main lexical items in Selected Headings.
[b] Based on individual totals of main lexical items in Selected Headings (see Table 40).
[c] Based on individual totals of nouns naming anatomical structures.
[d] Based on group totals of nouns naming anatomical structures.

Graph 53.

(a) *Nouns naming anatomical*
    structures: individual percentages

(b) *Nouns naming 'covert' anatomical*
    *structures: individual percentages**

(c) *Nouns naming 'overt' anatomical*
    *structures: individual percentages**

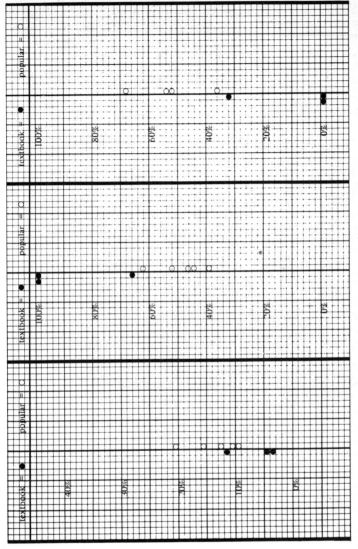

*Based on individual totals of nouns naming anatomical structures

Table 54.   *Distribution in Selected Headings of terms which belong to the domains of psychiatry, neurology, and behavioral psychology*

	T-1	T-2	T-3	Total	%[a]	P-1	P-2	P-3	P-4	P-5	Total	%[a]
	2	2	3	7	3	3	5	27	10	4	49	8
%[b]	2	3	5			4	4	12	11	5		

Table 55.   *Distribution in Selected Headings of terms which name certain sexual, social, and developmental states or roles of the human organism*

	T-1	T-2	T-3	Total	%[a]	P-1	P-2	P-3	P-4	P-5	Total	%[a]
	0	0	1	1	1	7	8	13	6	6	40	6
%[b]	0	0	2			10	4	6	8	7		

Table 56.   *Distribution in Selected Headings of terms which name so-called 'natural' approaches to the maintenance of health*

	T-1	T-2	T-3	Total	%[a]	P-1	P-2	P-3	P-4	P-5	Total	%[a]
	1	1	0	2	1	1	15	5	1	3	25	4
%[b]	1	1	0			1	11	2	1	4		

[a] Based on group totals of main lexical items in Selected Headings.
[b] Based on individual totals of main lexical items in Selected Headings (see Table 40).

iii.   *Objective no. three: A delineation of three taxonomic classes: Class T, Class P, and Class T ∩ P:* One of the consequences of having mapped the Selected Headings of the eight books of medical instruction onto the 'Categories' of the 'List of Three-digit Categories' was the formation of 16[27] different clusters or sets of semantically-related lexical items. The members of each of these 16 sets have been further divided (see Table 57 below) into three classes: Class T (exclusive to textbooks), Class P (exclusive to popular books) and Class T ∩ P (common to both). While it would be too strong a claim to say that those terms belonging to Classes P and T ∩ P are exemplative of medical terminology in current usage in popular speech, one could claim that the terms belonging to these two classes represent the editor or author's expectations concerning the familiarity of the reading public with such terminology.

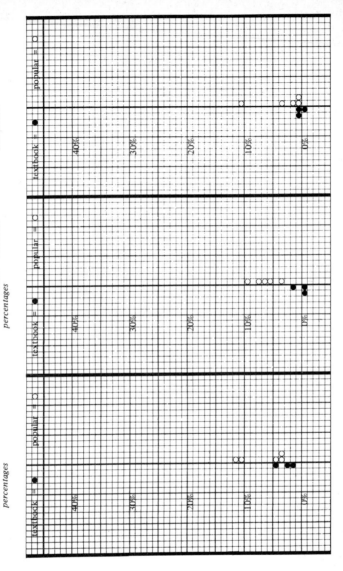

Graph 54. Terms which belong to the domains of psychiatry, neurology, and behavioral psychology: individual percentages

Graph 55. Terms which name certain sexual, social, and developmental states or roles of the human organism: individual percentages

Graph 56. Terms which name so-called 'natural' approaches to the maintenance of health: individual percentages

Table 57.   *Three taxonomic classes in Selected Headings*

'Category I: Infectious and Parasitic Diseases'

Class T:	Biological Agents
	Helminthic (Diseases)[a]
	Microbial (Diseases)
	Protozoan (Diseases)

Class P:	Amebiasis
	Boeck's Sarcoid
	Brucellosis
	Fevers
	Gonorrhea
	Hansen's Disease
	Hospital-caused (Infections)
	Infectious Mononucleosis
	Leprosy
	Malaria
	Nosocomial (Infections)
	Poliomyelitis
	Rabies
	Sarcoidosis
	Syphilis
	Tuberculosis
	Undulant Fever
	Venereal Diseases

Class T ∩ P:	Infections; Infectious

'Category II: Neoplasms'

Class T:	Neoplasia; Neoplastic (Diseases)

Class P:	Cancer
	Hodgkin's Disease

Class T ∩ P:	∅

'Category III: Endocrine, Nutritional and Metabolic Diseases, and Immunity Disorders'

Class T:	Electrolyte (Metabolism)
	Hormonal (Disorders)

contd.

[a] Bracketed words indicate the syntactic context.

Table 57 (*contd.*)

	Metabolic (Disorders); Metabolism (Disorders of) Water

Class P:

- Addison's Disease
- Adrenal Cortical Hyperfunction
- Allergies, Allergic (Disorders)
- Body Defences
- Cushing's Syndrome
- Diabetes
- Food
- Glands (Endocrine)
- Goiter
- Hay Fever
- Hypersensitivity
- Internal Secreting
- Male Climacteric
- Menopause
- Sex Life; Sexual (Disorders)
- Tonsillitis
- Vitamin Deficiencies
- Weight (Control), (Problems), (Loss and Gain of)

Class T ∩ P:

- Endocrine; Endocrinology
- Nutrition; Nutritional
- Immune; Immunity; Immunologic

'*Category IV: Diseases of the Blood and Blood-forming Organs*'

Class T:

- Hematopoietic (System), (Diseases)
- Hematologic (Diseases); Hematology

Class P:

- Anemia(s)
- Blood-forming Organs
- Hemophilia
- Leukemia
- Purpura

Class T ∩ P: 0

'*Category V: Mental Disorders*'

Class T: Behavior

contd.

Table 57 (*contd.*)

Class P: Emotional (Illness), (Disorders), (Development)
               Coping (Effectively)
               Mental (Illness), (Care), (Problems), (Stress), (Health)
               Mind
               Nervous (Disorders)
               Schizophrenia
               Senility
               Stress
               Tension

Class T ∩ P: Psychiatry; Psychiatric

'*Category VI: Diseases of the Nervous System and Sense Organs*'

Class T: Ophthalmology (in Medicine)

Class P: Brain
               Cerebral Palsy
               Dizziness
               Ears
               Epilepsy
               Eyes
               Headache
               Menieres Disease
               Migraine
               Motion Sickness
               Multiple Sclerosis
               Myasthenia Gravis
               Narcolepsy
               Nose
               Parkinson's Disease
               Sciatica
               Sense Organs
               Stroke
               Throat

Class T ∩ P: Nervous (System)

'*Category VII: Diseases of the Circulatory System*'

Class T: Cardiovascular (Diseases)
               Vascular (System)

contd.

Table 57 (*contd.*)

Class P: Blood Pressure (High), (Low)
              Blood Vessel (Diseases)
              Circulatory (System); Circulation
              Hemorrhoids
              Hypertension

Class T ∩ P: Heart

'*Category VIII: Diseases of the Respiratory System*'

Class T: Pulmonary (Disease)

Class P: Asthma
              Bronchitis
              Chest
              Colds
              Coughs
              Emphysema
              Flu
              Lungs
              Oxygen in the Body
              Pneumonias
              Sinusitis
              Sore Throats
              Tuberculosis

Class T ∩ P: Respiratory (System), (Disease), (Ailments)

'*Category IX: Diseases of the Digestive System*'

Class T: Alimentary Tract
              Gastrointestinal Tract
              Hepatobiliary (System)
              Pancreas

Class P: Appendix; Appendicitis
              Celiac (Disease)
              Colitis; Ulcerative Colitis
              Constipation
              Diarrhea
              Diverticulitis
              Gallstones

contd.

Table 57 (*contd.*)

	Hernia
	Ulcers (Peptic), (of Stomach), (of Duodenum)
Class T ∩ P:	Digestive (System), (Troubles), (Disturbances), (Ailments)
	Liver (Disease)

'*Category X: Diseases of the Genitourinary System'*

Class T:	Renal (Diseases), (Function)
	Urinary Tract

Class P:	Bedwetting
	Breast (Diseases)
	Fibroids
	Genitourinary (Tract), (System)
	Menopause
	Menstrual (Disorders)
	Prostate (Disorders)
	Special Concerns of Women

Class T ∩ P:	Kidneys; Kidney (Disease)

'*Category XI: Complications of Pregnancy, Childbirth, and the Puerperium'*

Class T:	∅

Class P:	Childbirth
	Miscarriage
	Pregnancy
	Toxemia (of Pregnancy)

Class T ∩ P:	∅

'*Category XII: Diseases of the Skin and Subcutaneous Tissue'*

Class T:	Cutaneous (Diseases), (Medicine)

Class P:	Hair
	Nails
	Psoriasis
	Scalp
	Shingles

contd.

Table 57 (*contd.*)

                Skin

Class T ∩ P: 0

'Category XIII: Diseases of the Musculoskeletal System and Connective Tissue'

Class T: (Bone) Mineral Metabolism
                Rheumatic (Disease)
                Rheumatoid (Arthritis)
                Striated (Muscle)

Class P: Arm
                Backache; Low Back Pain
                Bad Breath
                Body Mechanics
                Bruises
                Clubfoot
                Congenital Hip Dislocation
                Feet; Foot
                Gums
                Legs
                Muscular Dystrophy
                Neck
                Rheumatism
                Shoulder
                Skeletal (System)
                Sprains
                Strains
                Teeth
                Tetany

Class T ∩ P: Arthritis
                Bone
                Collagen (Diseases)
                Connective Tissue
                Joints
                Muscle

'Category XIV: Congenital Abnormalities'

Class T: Hereditary (Disorders)

contd.

Table 57 (*contd.*)

Class P:　　　Birth Defects
　　　　　　　Inheritance (of Disease)

Class T ∩ P:　Genetics; Genetic (Disorders), (Principles), (Problems)

'*Category XV: Certain Conditions Originating in the Perinatal Period*'

Class T:　　　∅

Class P:　　　Infant (Care)
　　　　　　　Child (Care)

Class T ∩ P:　∅

'*Category XVI: Symptoms, Signs, and Ill-defined Conditions*'

This Category will not be considered in this analysis because of a decision to map all terms for specific signs and symptoms on to those 'Categories' with which they are most frequently identified. See note[b] in Supplement B-1(a), p. 144.

'*Category XVII: Injury and Poisoning*'

Class T:　　　(Disorders Due to) Chemical Agents
　　　　　　　Environmental Factors
　　　　　　　Medical Emergencies

Class P:　　　First Aid
　　　　　　　Food Poisoning
　　　　　　　Home Accidents
　　　　　　　Insect Pests
　　　　　　　Poisoning
　　　　　　　Rabies
　　　　　　　(The) Inhaling of Dangerous Substances

Class T ∩ P:　Physical (Agents), (Forces)

To summarize:

　The Selected Headings of the Tables of Contents of the eight books of medical instruction have been investigated with three objectives in mind:

1. To compare the broad scope of textbooks vs popular books.

2. To determine how textbooks differ from popular books with respect to the linguistic properties of their Selected Headings, the assumption being that such properties of the Selected Headings are likely to be representative of the properties of lexical items distributed throughout the Texts.

3. To identify, according to the 'List of Three-digit Categories', 16 sets of semantically-related lexical items, and to delineate the members of each of these sets into three taxonomic classes: Class T (exclusive to textbooks), Class P (exclusive to popular books), and Class T ∩ P (common to both).

All data appearing in the various Tables in the foregoing section, and in their companion Graphs, and in their corresponding Supplements will be cited in Part Three as evidence pointing to the ways in which textbooks differ from popular books with respect to their form and contents.

Having investigated the Texts and the Tables of Contents of the selected books, we will then turn to the third and final 'segment', namely, the Paratext.

SUPPLEMENT B

B-1 (a) *Mapping Procedure Between Selected Headings and the 'List of Three-digit Categories':*

(i) *Textbooks*

List of Three-digit Categories	Selected Heading (T-1)
I. Infectious and Parasitic Diseases	Part 6: Disorders Caused by Biologic Agents
II. Neoplasms	Part 7: (S9[a]): Neoplasia
III. Endocrine, Nutritional, and Metabolic Diseases, and Immunity Disorders	Part 4: Nutritional, Hormonal, and Metabolic Disorders
	Part 3: (S3) : Metabolic Considerations
	Part 3: (S4) : Immunologic Considerations

contd.

B-1 (a), (i) Textbooks (*contd.*)

List of Three-digit Categories	Selected Heading (T-1)
IV. Diseases of the Blood and Blood-forming Organs	Part 7: (S8) : Disorders of the Hematopoietic System
V. Mental Disorders	Part 7: (S11): Psychiatric Disorders
VI. Diseases of the Nervous System and Sense Organs	Part 7: (S10): Disorders of the Nervous System
VII. Diseases of the Circulatory System	Part 7: (S1) : Disorders of the Heart Part 7: (S2) : Disorders of the Vascular System
VIII. Diseases of the Respiratory System	Part 7: (S3) : Disorders of the Respiratory System
IX. Diseases of the Digestive System	Part 7: (S5) : Disorders of the Alimentary Tract Part 7: (S6) : Disorders of the Hepatobiliary System Part 7: (S7) : Disorders of the Pancreas
X. Diseases of the Genito-urinary System	Part 7: (S4) : Diseases of the Kidneys and Urinary Tract
XI. Complications of Pregnancy, Childbirth, and the Puerperium	———
XII. Diseases of the Skin and Subcutaneous Tissue	———
XIII. Diseases of the Musculo-skeletal System and Connective Tissue	Part 7: (S12): Diseases of the Striated Muscle Part 7: (S13): Disorders of Bone and Bone Mineral Metabolism

contd.

B-1 (a), (i) Textbooks (*contd.*)

List of Three-digit Categories	Selected Heading (T-1)
	Part 7: (S14): Disorders of Joints and Connective Tissues
XIV. Congenital Anomalies	Part 3: (S1) : Genetics and Human Disease Part 7: (S15): Genetic Disorders of Supporting Tissues
XV. Certain Conditions Originating in the Perinatal Period	———
XVI. Symptoms, Signs, and Ill-defined Conditions	Part 2: Cardinal Manifestations and Approach to Disease
XVII. Injury and Poisoning	Part 5: Disorders due to Chemical and Physical Agents

[a] Section.

List of Three-digit Categories	Selected Heading (T-2)
I. Infectious and Parasitic Diseases	Part 8: [a]Microbial Diseases Part 9: Protozoan and Helminthic Diseases
II. Neoplasms	———
III. Endocrine, Nutritional, and Metabolic Diseases, and Immunity Disorders	Part 18: Diseases of the Endocrine System Part 15: Diseases of Nutrition Part 17: Diseases of Metabolism Part 4: Immune Disease
IV. Diseases of the Blood and Blood-forming Disorders	Part 16: Hematologic and Hematopoietic Diseases
V. Mental Disorders	Part 10: Disorders of the Nervous System and Behavior

contd.

B-1 (a), (i) Textbooks (*contd.*)

List of Three-digit Categories	Selected Heading (T-2)
VI. Diseases of the Nervous System and Sense Organs	
VII. Diseases of the Circulatory System	Part 12: Cardiovascular Diseases
VIII. Diseases of the Respiratory System	Part 11: Respiratory Diseases
IX. Diseases of the Digestive System	Part 14: Diseases of the Digestive System
X. Diseases of the Genitourinary System	Part 13: Renal Diseases
XI. Complications of Pregnancy, Childbirth, and the Puerperium	——
XII. Diseases of the Skin and Subcutaneous Tissue	Part 20: Certain Cutaneous Diseases with Significant Systemic Manifestations
XIII. Diseases of the Musculoskeletal System and Connective Tissue	Part 19: Diseases of Bone Part 6: Diseases of the Joints Part 5: Connective Tissue Diseases ('Collagen Diseases') other than Rheumatoid Arthritis
XIV. Congenital Anomalies	Part 2: Genetic Principles Part 21: Miscellaneous Hereditary Disorders Affecting Multiple Organ Systems
XV. Certain Conditions Originating in the Perinatal Period	——
XVI. Symptoms, Signs, and Ill-defined Conditions	——

contd.

B-1 (a), (i) Textbooks (*contd.*)

List of Three-digit Categories	Selected Headings (T-2)
XVII. Injury and Poisoning	Part 3: Environmental Factors in Disease

[a] Because of space restrictions, Arabic numerals (rather than the original Roman numerals) have been used to indicate the Parts of this book.

List of Three-digit Categories	Selected Heading (T-3)
I. Infectious and Parasitic Diseases	[a]S-12: Infectious Diseases
II. Neoplasms	S-8 : Neoplastic Diseases
III. Endocrine, Nutritional, and Metabolic Diseases, and Immunity Disorders	S-11: Endocrinology S-2 : Disorders of Water and Electrolyte Metabolism S-13: Diseases with Abnormalities of Immunity
IV. Diseases of the Blood and Blood-forming Organs	S-7 : Hematology
V. Mental Disorders	S-16: Psychiatry in Medicine
VI. Diseases of the Nervous System and Sense Organs	S-15: Disorders of the Nervous System S-19 (163): Ophthalmology in Medicine
VII. Diseases of the Circulatory System	S-4 : Cardiovascular Disease
VIII. Diseases of the Respiratory System	S-5 : Pulmonary Disease
IX. Diseases of the Digestive System	S-9 : Diseases of the Gastrointestinal Tract S-10: Diseases of the Liver
X. Diseases of the Genitourinary System	S-3 : Renal Diseases and Disturbances in Renal Function

contd.

B-1 (a), (i) Textbooks (*contd.*)

List of Three-digit Categories	Selected Heading (T-3)
XI. Complications of Pregnancy, Childbirth, and the Puerperium	
XII. Diseases of the Skin and Subcutaneous Tissue	S-19 (164): Cutaneous Medicine
XIII. Diseases of the Musculoskeletal System and Connective Tissue	S-14: Rheumatic Disease
XIV. Congenital Anomalies	S-6 : Medical Genetics
XV. Certain Conditions Originating in the Perinatal Period	
XVI. Symptoms, Signs and Ill-defined Conditions	
XVII. Injury and Poisoning	S-18: Medical Emergencies

[a] Section.

(ii) *Popular books*

List of Three-digit Categories	Selected Heading (P-1)
I. Infectious and Parasitic Diseases	Ch.[a] 2 : Infectious Diseases
II. Neoplasms	Ch. 26: Cancer
III. Endocrine, Nutritional, and Metabolic Diseases, and Immunity Disorders	Ch. 9 : The Endocrine Glands Ch. 14: Nutrition Ch. 20: Allergies and Hypersensitivity
IV. Diseases of the Blood and Blood-forming Organs	Ch. 4 : Blood-forming Organs and their Disorders

contd.

B-1 (a), (ii) Popular books (*contd.*)

List of Three-digit Categories	Selected Heading (P-1)
V. Mental Disorders	Ch. 21: Emotional and Mental Illness
VI. Diseases of the Nervous System and Sense Organs	Ch. 7 : The Nervous System Ch. 16: The Eyes Ch. 17: The Ears, Nose, and Throat
VII. Diseases of the Circulatory System	Ch. 3 : The Heart and Circulatory System
VIII. Diseases of the Respiratory System	Ch. 6 : The Lungs and Chest in Health and Disease
IX. Diseases of the Digestive System	Ch. 13: The Digestive System
X. Diseases of the Genitourinary System	Ch. 8 : Kidneys and the Genitourinary System Ch. 12: Special Concerns of Women
XI. Complications of Pregnancy, Childbirth, and the Puerperium	Ch. 10: Pregnancy and Childbirth
XII. Diseases of the Skin and Subcutaneous Tissue	Ch. 5 : The Skin and its Disorders
XIII. Diseases of the Musculoskeletal System and Connective Tissue	Ch. 15: The Teeth and their Care Ch. 18: Bones, Muscles and their Disorders Ch. 19: Arthritis and Rheumatism
XIV. Congenital Anomalies	Ch. 15: Medical Genetics
XV. Certain Conditions Originating in the Perinatal Period	Ch. 11: Infant and Child Care
XVI. Symptoms, Signs, and Ill-defined Conditions	(see note b, p. 144)

contd.

B-1 (a), (ii) Popular books (*contd.*)

List of Three-digit Categories	Selected Heading (P-1)
XVII.　Injury and Poisoning	Ch.　28: First Aid for Your Family

[a] Chapter.

[b] Certain difficulties arose in relation to Category XVI: 'Symptoms, Signs and Ill-defined Conditions'. Whereas lexical items referring to specific signs or symptoms (e.g. 'cough', 'backache', etc.) were entirely absent from the Selected Headings of textbooks (although T-1 does have a Selected Heading called 'Cardinal Manifestations and Approach to Disease'), such lexical items appeared with frequency in the Selected Headings of popular books. A question arose as to whether such lexical items should be mapped on to Category XVI, or, instead, upon another 'Category' which indicated a certain class of disorders with which that sign or symptom is usually associated (in which case, the items 'cough' and 'backache' would be mapped, respectively, upon Category IV: 'Diseases of the Respiratory System', and Category XIII: 'Diseases of the Musculoskeletal System and Connective Tissue'. Although neither alternative was entirely satisfactory, a decision was made to opt for the second choice, since it enabled the writer to bring into contiguity a greater number of semantically-related lexical items, and facilitated a subsequent division of all main lexical items appearing in Selected Headings into three classes: Class T (exclusive to textbooks), Class P (exclusive to popular books), and Class T ∩ P (common to both).

List of Three-digit Categories	Selected Heading (P-2)
I.　Infectious and Parasitic Diseases	
II.　Neoplasms	
III.　Endocrine, Nutritional, and Metabolic Diseases, and Immunity Disorders	14. How to Boost Your Sex Life and Ease the Strain of the Menopause and the Male Climacteric
IV.　Diseases of the Blood and Blood-forming Organs	
V.　Mental Disorders	3. How to Cope with Disease More Successfully by Relieving Everyday Stress and Tension with Naturomatic Healing

contd.

B-1 (a), (ii) Popular books (*contd.*)

List of Three-digit Categories	Selected Heading (P-2)
VI. Diseases of the Nervous System and Sense Organs	
VII. Diseases of the Circulatory System	1. How to Extend Your Life with Naturomatic Healing of Heart and Blood Vessel Disease
VIII. Diseases of the Respiratory System	2. Naturomatic Healing Methods for Coughs, Colds, Sore Throats, and Other Respiratory Ailments
IX. Diseases of the Digestive System	8. Tested Naturomatic Healing Methods for Headache, Constipation, and Hemorrhoids 9. How to Relieve the Pain and Misery of Stomach Ulcers, Colitis, and other Digestive Troubles with Naturomatic Healing
X. Diseases of the Genito-urinary System	
XI. Complications of Pregnancy, Childbirth, and the Puerperium	
XII. Diseases of the Skin and Subcutaneous Tissue	11. How to Treat Simple Skin Disorders with Naturomatic Healing
XIII. Diseases of the Musculo-skeletal System and Connective Tissue	4. How to Relieve Daily Aches and Pains with Good Body Mechanics and Proper Foot Care 5. First Aid Nature's Way for Bruises, Strains, Sprains, and Muscle Injuries 6. How to Relieve Neck, Arm, and Shoulder Pain with Drug-

contd.

B-1 (a), (ii) Popular books (*contd.*)

List of Three-digit Categories	Selected Heading (P-2)
	less Methods of Naturomatic Healing
	7. How to get Prompt Relief from Backache, Arthritis, and Leg Pain with Naturomatic Healing
	10. How to Care for Your Teeth, Gums, Bones, and Joints with Naturomatic Healing Methods
XIV. Congenital Anomalies	
XV. Certain Conditions Originating in the Perinatal Period	
XVI. Symptoms, Signs and Ill-defined Conditions	(see note b, p. 144)
XVII. Injury and Poisoning	15. Miscellaneous Naturomatic Remedies for a Variety of Injuries and Ailments

List of Three-digit Categories	Selected Heading (P-3)
I. Infectious and Parasitic Diseases	DS[a] 4: Amebiasis
	DS 13: Brucellosis (Undulant Fever)
	DS 24: Gonorrhea and Other Venereal Diseases
	DS 33: Leprosy (Hansen's Disease)
	DS 37: Malaria
	DS 40: Infectious Mononucleosis
	DS 48: Poliomyelitis
	DS 52: Sarcoidosis (Boeck's Sarcoid)
	DS 59: Syphilis
	DS 60: Tuberculosis
II. Neoplasms	DS 15: Cancer
	DS 31: Hodgkin's Disease

contd.

B-1 (a), (ii) Popular books (*contd.*)

List of Three-digit Categories	Selected Heading (P-3)
III. Endocrine, Nutritional, and Metabolic Diseases, and Immunity Disorders	Part 2 (6): The Food You Eat Part 3 (25): The Endocrine Glands Part 3 (28): Body Defences and Medical Reinforcements DS 1: Addison's Disease DS 3: Allergy DS 19: Cushing's Syndrome (Adrenal Cortical Hyperfunction) DS 20: Diabetes
IV. Diseases of the Blood and Blood-forming Organs	DS 5: Anemias DS 27: Hemophilia and Related Diseases DS 34: Leukemia DS 51: Purpura
V. Mental Disorders	Part 4 (29): Mind, Body, Mind Part 4 (30): The Guises of Mental Problems Part 4 (31): Coping Effectively Part 4 (32): Help for Emotional Problems Part 4 (33): Other Problems, Other Helps Part 4 (34): Preventive Psychiatry DS[a] 53: Schizophrenia DS 55: Senility
VI. Diseases of the Nervous System and Sense Organs	Part 3 (23): The Brain and Nervous System Part 3 (24): The Sense Organs DS 16: Cerebral Palsy DS 21: Dizziness and Menieres Disease DS 22: Epilepsy DS 25: Headache (Including Migraine) DS 41: Motion Sickness DS 42: Multiple Sclerosis

contd.

B-1 (a), (ii) Popular books (*contd.*)

List of Three-digit Categories	Selected Heading (P-3)
	DS 44: Myasthenia Gravis
	DS 45: Narcolepsy (and Related Conditions)
	DS 46: Parkinson's Disease
	DS 54: Sciatica
	DS 57: Stroke
VII. Diseases of the Circulatory System	Part 3 (19): The Circulatory System
	DS 26: Heart Diseases
	DS 28: Hemorrhoids
	DS 30: High Blood Pressure (Hypertension)
	DS 36: Low Blood Pressure
	DS 63: Varicose Veins
VIII. Diseases of the Respiratory System	Part 3 (20): The Respiratory System
	DS 8: Asthma
	DS 12: Chronic Bronchitis and Emphysema
	DS 18: Common Cold
	DS 47: The Pneumonias
	DS 56: Sinusitis (Acute and Chronic)
IX. Diseases of the Digestive System	Part 3 (21): The Digestive System
	DS 6: Appendicitis
	DS 23: Gallbladder Disease
	DS 29: Hernia
	DS 35: Liver Disease
	DS 61: Ulcer of the Stomach and Duodenum (Peptic Ulcer)
	DS 62: Ulcerative Colitis
X. Diseases of the Genito-urinary System	Part 3 (22): The Genitourinary System
	DS 11: Breast Diseases
	DS 32: Kidney Disease
	DS 38: Menopause

contd.

B-1 (a), (ii) Popular books (*contd.*)

List of Three-digit Categories	Selected Heading (P-3)
	DS 39: Menstrual Disorders and Fibroids
	49: Prostate Gland Enlargement
XI. Complications of Pregnancy, Childbirth, and the Puerperium	
XII. Diseases of the Skin and Subcutaneous Tissue	Part 3 (16): The Skin, Hair, and Nails
	DS 50: Psoriasis
XIII. Diseases of the Musculo-skeletal System and Connective Tissue	Part 3 (17): The Skeletal System
	Part 3 (18): The Muscles
	Part 3 (26): The Teeth
	Part 3 (27): The Feet
	DS 7: Arthritis
	DS 9: Low Back Pain
	DS 10: Bone Disease
	DS 14: Bursitis
	DS 17: Clubfoot and Congenital Hip Dislocation
	DS 43: Muscle Disorders
XIV. Congenital Anomalies	Part 5 (38): Genetic Problems and Counseling
XV. Certain Conditions Originating in the Perinatal Period	
XVI. Symptoms, Signs, and Ill-defined Conditions	(see note b, p. 144)
XVII. Injury and Poisoning	Part 5 (40): Home Accidents and their Prevention

^a *Disease Scenarios.*

B-1 (a), (ii) Popular books (*contd.*)

List of Three-digit Categories	Selected Heading (P-4)
I. Infections and Parasitic Diseases	39. Hospital-Caused (nosocomial) Infections 44. Mononucleosis 50. Rabies 62. Venereal Diseases
II. Neoplasms	13. Cancer
III. Endocrine, Nutritional, and Metabolic Diseases, and Immunity Disorders	2. Allergy 19. Diabetes 32. Goiter 34. Hay Fever 51. Sexual Disorders 57. Tonsillitis 63. Weight Problems
IV. Diseases of the Blood and Blood-forming Organs	3. Anemia
V. Mental Disorders	24. Emotional and Nervous Disorders
VI. Diseases of the Nervous System and Sense Organs	23. The Ears and Hearing 26. Epilepsy 27. The Eyes 35. Headache 45. Motion Sickness 46. Multiple Sclerosis 47. Muscular Dystrophy 48. Parkinson's Disease
VII. Diseases of the Circulatory System	16. Circulation 36. The Heart 37. Hemorrhoids 61. Varicose Veins
VIII. Diseases of the Respiratory System	6. Asthma 12. Bronchitis 17. Colds 25. Emphysema

contd.

B-1 (a), (ii) Popular books (*contd.*)

List of Three-digit Categories	Selected Heading (P-4)
	29. Flu
	53. Sinusitis
	59. Tuberculosis
IX. Diseases of the Digestive System	4. The Appendix
	14. Celiac Disease
	18. Constipation
	20. Diarrhea
	21. Digestive System Ailments
	22. Diverticulitis
	31. Gallstones
	38. Hernia
	42. The Liver
	60. Ulcers
X. Diseases of the Genito-urinary System	9. Bedwetting
	41. Kidney Disease
	49. Prostate Disorders
XI. Complications of Pregnancy, Childbirth, and the Puerperium	43. Miscarriage
	58. Toxemia of Pregnancy
XII. Diseases of the Skin and Subcutaneous Tissue	33. Hair and Scalp Problems
	52. Shingles
	54. The Skin
XIII. Diseases of the Musculo-skeletal System and Connective Tissue	2. Bad Breath
	5. Arthritis
	7. Backache
	11. Bone Diseases
	28. Feet
	55. Avoiding Ailments of Teeth and Gums
	56. Tetany
XIV. Congenital Anomalies	10. Birth Defects
XV. Certain Conditions Originating in the Perinatal Period	⎯⎯

contd.

B-1 (a), (ii) Popular books (*contd.*)

List of Three-digit Categories	Selected Heading (P-4)
XVI. Symptoms, Signs, and Ill-defined Conditions	(see note b, p. 144)
XVII. Injury and Poisoning	30. Food Poisoning

List of Three-digit Categories	Selected Heading (P-5)
I. Infectious and Parasitic Diseases	21. Fevers and Infections 27. The Venereal Diseases
II. Neoplasms	24. Cancer
III. Endocrine, Nutritional, and Metabolic Diseases, and Immunity Disorders	12. Allergic Disorders 14. Loss and Gain of Weight 15. Vitamin Deficiencies 16. The Internal Secreting or Endocrine Glands 22. Infections and Immunity
IV. Diseases of the Blood and Blood-forming Organs	
V. Mental Disorders	11. Emotional Development and Mental Stress 30. Mental Health
VI. Diseases of the Nervous System and Sense Organs	25. Eyes 26. Nose, Throat, and Ear
VII. Diseases of the Circulatory System	5. Blood Pressure 6. Your Heart and Circulation
VIII. Diseases of the Respiratory System	4. Oxygen in the Body
IX. Diseases of the Digestive System	7. Digestive Disturbances

contd.

B-1 (a), (ii) Popular books (*contd.*)

List of Three-digit Categories	Selected Heading (P-5)
X. Diseases of the Genito-urinary System	8. The Kidneys
XI. Complications of Pregnancy, Childbirth, and the Puerperium	
XII. Diseases of the Skin and Subcutaneous Tissue	23. Some Common Skin Diseases
XIII. Diseases of the Musculo-skeletal System and Connective Tissue	13. Diseases of Connective Tissue—Collagen Disease 17. Disorders of Bones 28. The Care of the Feet
XIV. Congenital Anomalies	9. Inheritance of Disease
XV. Certain Conditions Originating in the Perinatal Period	
XVI. Symptoms, Signs, and Ill-defined Conditions	2. Symptoms of Disease 3. Understanding Symptoms
XVII. Injury and Poisoning	18. Poisoning 19. Effects of Physical Forces on the Body 20. The Inhaling of Dangerous Substances 29. Insect Pests 34. First Aid and Common Complaints

B-1 (b)
'Leftover' Selected Headings

(i)   *Textbooks*

T-1
Part One: The Physician and the Patient

B-1 (b) (*contd.*)

Part Three,
    Section 2:   Clinical Pharmacology

T-2
Part   I: The Nature of Medicine
Part   VII: Granulomatous Diseases of Unproved Etiology
Part XXII: Normal Laboratory Values of Clinical Importance

T-3
Section One: The Approach to the Patient
Section Seventeen: Diseases of Medical Management
Section Nineteen,
    161:                 Medical Problems Associated with Alcoholism
Section Nineteen,
    162:                 Adolescent Medicine

(ii)   *Popular books*

P-1
Chapter 1:   Home Care of the Patient
Chapter 22:   Your Operation
Chapter 23:   X-Rays and You
Chapter 24:   Laboratory Tests
Chapter 27:   Drug Use and Abuse

P-2
        12:             How to Relieve Fatigue and Rejuvenate Your Body
                        with Massage and Naturomatic Tonics
        13:             How to Reverse the Causes of Premature Aging and
                        Remain Younger Longer with Naturomatic Healing

P-3
Part Two,   8:   Physical Activity
Part Two,   9:   Sleep
Part Two,   10:   Relaxation
Part Two,   11:   Smoking
Part Two,   12:   Drinking
Part Two,   13:   Drugs
Part Two,   14:   Your Work and Your Health
Part Three, 15:   The Basic Strengths of the Human Body
Part Five,   35:   Healthy Adjustment in Marriage
Part Five,   36:   Sexual Adjustment in Marriage

B-1 (b) (*contd.*)

B-1 (c)
Unmapped 'Categories'

'Category'[a]		Where Absent
I. Infectious and Parasitic Diseases		P-2
II. Neoplasms	T-2	P-2
*III. Endocrine, Nutritional, and Metabolic Diseases, and Immunity Disorders		
IV. Diseases of the Blood and Blood-forming Organs		P-2 P-5
*V. Mental Disorders		
VI. Diseases of the Nervous System and Sense Organs		P-2
*VII. Diseases of the Circulatory System		
*VIII. Diseases of the Respiratory System		

contd.

B-1 (c) (*contd.*)

'Category'[a]	Where Absent	
*IX. Diseases of the Digestive System		
X. Diseases of the Genitourinary System		P-2
XI. Complications of Pregnancy, Childbirth, and the Puerperium	T-1 T-2 T-3	P-2 P-3 P-5
XII. Diseases of the Skin and Subcutaneous Tissue	T-1	
*XIII. Diseases of the Musculoskeletal System and Connective Tissue		
XIV. Congenital Anomalies		P-2
XV. Certain Conditons Originating in the Perinatal Period	T-1 T-2 T-3	P-2 P-3 P-4 P-5
XVI. Symptoms, Signs, and Ill-defined Conditions	T-2 T-3	P-1
*XVII. Injury and Poisoning		

[a]   Those items marked * indicate 'Categories' for which corresponding Selected Headings exist in *all* textbooks and *all* popular books investigated in this study.

B-2
Main Lexical Items[a] *in the 'List of Three-digit Categories'*[b]

infectious	complications
parasitic	pregnancy
diseases (10)[c]	childbirth
neoplasms	puerperium
endocrine	skin
	subcutaneous

contd.

B-2 (*contd.*)

nutritional
metabolic
immunity
disorders (2)
blood
blood-forming
organs (2)
mental
nervous
system (6)
sense
circulatory
respiratory
digestive
genitourinary

tissue (2)
musculoskeletal
connective
congenital
anomalies
certain
conditions (2)
originating
perinatal
period
symptoms
signs
ill-defined
injury
poisoning

---

[a] As indicated earlier (Part Two, Section I: 5), main lexical items include all words with the exception of articles, prepositions, and conjunctions.
[b] Hereafter indicated simply as the 'List'.
[c] Bracketed numbers indicate frequency of occurrence.

B-3
Basic List of Main Lexical Items in Selected Headings

T-1	T-2
physician (2)[a]	nature
patient	medicine
cardinal	genetic
manifestations	principles
approach (2)	environmental
disease(s) (4)	factor
biological	disease(s) (18)
considerations (3)	immune
clinical (2)	connective
medicine	tissue
genetics	collagen
human	rheumatoid
pharmacology	arthritis
metabolic (2)	joints
immunologic	granulomatous

contd.

B-3 (*contd.*)

T-1	T-2
nutritional	unproved
hormonal	etiology
disorders (16)	microbial
due	protozoan
chemical	helminthic
physical	disorders (2)
agents (2)	nervous
caused	system(s) (4)
biologic	behavior
organ	respiratory
system(s) (6)	cardiovascular
heart	renal
vascular	digestive
respiratory	nutrition
kidneys	hematologic
urinary	hematopoietic
tract (2)	metabolism
alimentary	endocrine
hepatobiliary	bone
pancreas	certain
hematopoietic	cutaneous
neoplasia	significant
nervous	systemic
psychiatric	manifestations
striated	miscellaneous
muscle	hereditary
bone (2)	affecting
mineral	multiple
metabolism	organ
joints	normal
connective	laboratory
tissue(s) (2)	values
genetic	clinical
supporting	importance
Total = 82	Total = 70

B-3 (*contd.*)

T-3	P-1
approach	home
patient	care (3)
disorders (2)	patient
water	infectious
electrolyte	disease(s) (2)
metabolism	heart
renal (2)	circulatory
disease(s) (10)	system (3)
disturbances	blood-forming
function	organs
cardiovascular	their (3)
pulmonary	disorders (3)
medical (4)	skin
genetics	its
hematology	lungs
neoplastic	chest
gastrointestinal	health
tract	nervous
liver	kidneys
endocrinology	genitourinary
infectious	tract
abnormalities	endocrine
immunity	glands
rheumatic	pregnancy
nervous	childbirth
system	infant
psychiatry	child
medicine (5)	special
management	concerns
emergencies	women
special	digestive
topics	nutrition
problems	teeth
associated	eyes
alcoholism	ears
adolescent	nose
ophthalmology	throat
cutaneous	bones
Total = 56	muscles
	arthritis

contd.

B-3 (*contd.*)

	P-1
	rheumatism
	allergies
	hypersensitivity
	emotional
	mental
	illness
	your (2)
	operation
	X-rays
	you
	laboratory
	tests
	medical
	genetics
	cancer
	drug
	use
	abuse
	first
	aid
	family
	Total = 71

P-2

how (11)	body (2)	colitis
to extend	mechanics	digestive
your (4)	proper	troubles
life (2)	foot	teeth
naturomatic (12)	care (2)	gums
healing (10)	first	bones
heart	aid	joints
blood	nature's	to treat
vessel	way	simple
disease(s) (2)	bruises	skin
methods (4)	strain(s) (2)	disorders
coughs	sprains	fatigue
colds	muscle	rejuvenate

contd.

B-3 (*contd.*)

P-2

sore	injuries (2)	massage
throat	neck	tonics
other (2)	arm	to reverse
respiratory	shoulder	causes
ailments (2)	drugless	premature
to cope	to get	aging
more	prompt	remain
successfully	relief	younger
relieving	backache	longer
everyday	arthritis	to boost
stress	leg	sex
tension	tested	ease
to relieve (4)	headache	menopause
daily	constipation	male
aches	hemorrhoids	climacteric
pain(s) (4)	misery	miscellaneous
good	stomach	remedies
	ulcers	variety
		Total = 142

P-3

promise	teeth	chronic	liver (2)
nature	feet	bronchitis	malaria
preventive (7)	defences	emphysema	menopause
prevention (1)	medical	brucellosis	menstrual
medicine (2)	reinforcements	undulant	disorders (2)
building	mental (2)	fever	fibroids
general	mind (2)	bursitis	infectious
health (2)	guises	cancer	mononucleosis
healthy (2)	problems (4)	cerebral	motion
therapy	coping	palsy	sickness
foods	effectively	clubfoot	multiple
you	help	congenital	sclerosis
eat	emotional	hip	myasthenia
weight	other (3)	dislocation	gravis
control	helps	common	narcolepsy
physical	psychitary	cold	related

contd.

B-3 (*contd.*)

P-3

activity	family	Cushing's	conditions
sleep	adjustment (2)	syndrome	Parkinson's
relaxation	marriage (2)	adrenal	pneumonias
smoking	sexual	cortical	poliomyelitis
drinking	toward	hyperfunction	prostate
drugs	parenthood	diabetes	gland
your (2)	genetic	dizziness	enlargement
work	counseling	Meniere's	psoriasis
body (4)	children	epilepsy	purpura
care (3)	home	gallbladder	sarcoidosis
basic	accidents	gonorrhea	Boeck's
strengths	their	venereal	sarcoid
human	diseases (15)	headache	schizophrenia
skin	scenarios	including	sciatica
hair	Addison's	migraine	senility
nails	. aging	heart	sinuses
skeletal	allergy	hemophilia	acute
system (6)	amebiasis	related	chronic
muscle(s) (2)	amebic (2)	hemorrhoids	stroke
circulatory	dysentery	hernia	suicide
respiratory	anemias	high	syphilis
digestive	appendicitis	blood (2)	tuberculosis
genitourinary	arthritis	pressure (2)	ulcer (2)
brain	asthma	hypertension	stomach
nervous	low (2)	Hodgkin's	duodenum
sense	back	kidney	peptic
organs	pain	leprosy	ulcerative
endocrine	bone	Hansen's	colitis
glands	. breast	leukemia	varicose
			veins
			Total = 232

P-4

alcoholism	scalp
allergy	problems (2)
anemia	hay
appendix	fever

P-5

when	secreting
you	endocrine
see	glands
doctor	bones

contd.

B-3 (*contd.*)

P-4 (*contd.*)		P-5 (*contd.*)	
arthritis	headache	symptoms (2)	poisoning
asthma	heart	disease(s) (6)	effects
backache	hemorrhoids	understanding	physical
bad	hernia	oxygen	forces
breath	hospital-caused	body (3)	inhaling
bedwetting	nosocomial	blood	dangerous
birth	infections	pressure	substances
defects	insomnia	your (2)	fevers
bone	kidney	heart	infections (2)
disease(s) (6)	liver	circulation	immunity
bronchitis	miscarriage	digestive	common (2)
cancer	mononucleosis	disturbances	skin
celiac	motion	kidneys	cancer
childhood	sickness	inheritance	eyes
circulation	multiple	aging	nose
colds	sclerosis	breakdown	throat
constipation	muscular	emotional	ear
diabetes	dystrophy	development	venereal
diarrhea	Parkinson's	mental (2)	care
digestive	prostate	stress	feet
system	rabies	allergic	insect
ailments (2)	sexual	disorders (2)	pests
diverticulitis	shingles	connective	health
ears	sinusitis	tissue	family
hearing	skin	collagen	medicine
emotional	avoiding	loss	chest
nervous	teeth	gain	exercise
disorders (3)	gums	weight	vacation
emphysema	tetany	vitamin	first
epilepsy	tonsillitis	deficiencies	aid
eyes	toxemia	internal	complaints
feet	pregnancy		
flu	tuberculosis		
food	ulcers		
poisoning	varicose		
gallstones	veins		
goiter	venereal		
hair	weight		
	Total = 93		Total = 84

[a] Bracketed numbers indicate frequency of occurrence.

B-4

Selected Headings: Monosyllabic Words (Table 41, Graph 41)

The 'List'	your (2)	treat	high	P-5
blood	you	skin	blood	when
sense	tests	boost	Boeck's	you
skin	drug	sex	stroke	see
signs	use	ease	veins	blood
	first	male		your (2)
T-1	aid		P-4	heart
due		P-3	bad	stress
caused	P-2	health (2)	breath	loss
heart	how (11)	foot	birth	gain
tract (2)[a]	your (4)	you	bone	weight
bone (2)	pain(s) (4)	eat	colds	glands
joints	life (2)	weight	ears	bones
	heart	sleep	eyes	skin
T-2	blood	drugs	feet	eyes
joints	coughs	your (2)	flu	nose
bone	colds	work	flood	throat
	sore	care (3)	hair	ear
T-3	throat	strengths	scalp	care
tract	cope	skin	hay	feet
	more	hair	heart	pests
P-1	stress	nails	skin	health
home	aches	brain	teeth	chest
care (3)	good	sense	gums	first
heart	foot	gland(s) (2)	veins	aid
skin	care (2)	teeth	weight	
its	first	feet		
lungs	aid	mind (2)		
chest	way	help		
health	strain(s) (2)	helps		
tract	sprains	home		
glands	neck	their		
child	arm	low (2)		
teeth	get	back		
eyes	prompt	pain		
ears	leg	bone		
nose	teeth	breast		
throat	gums	hip		
bones	bones	cold		
their (3)	joints	heart		

[a] Bracketed numbers indicate frequency of occurrence.

B-5 *Selected Headings: Personal Pronouns* (Table 42, Graph 42)	B-6 *Selected Headings: Gerunds* (Table 43, Graph 43)
The 'List' 0	*The 'List'* poisoning
T-1 0	*T-1* 0
T-2 0	*T-2* 0
T-3 0	*T-3* 0
P-1 their (3)* its your (2) you	*P-1* 0
P-2 your (4)	*P-2* healing (10) relieving aging
P-3 you your (2) their	*P-3* building smoking drinking coping counseling
P-4 0	*P-4* bed-wetting hearing poisoning avoiding

contd.

B-5 (*contd.*)   B-6 (*contd.*)

P-5   *P-5*
you   understanding
your (2)   aging
                                        poisoning
                                        inhaling

* Bracketed numbers indicate frequency of occurence.

B-7
Selected Headings: Compound Nouns[a] (Table 44, Graph 44)

The 'List'
immunity disorders
sense organs

T-1
human diseases
chemical agents
organ systems
bone mineral metabolism

T-2
(connective)[b] tissue diseases
collagen diseases
organ systems
laboratory values

T-3
electrolyte metabolism
adolescent medicine

P-1
home care
child care
laboratory tests
drug use

P-2
blood vessel diseases
healing methods (2)[c]
body mechanics
foot care
muscle injuries
shoulder pain
backache
leg pain
stomach ulcers
skin disorders
sex life
male climacteric

P-3
weight control
body care
human body
sense organs
body defences
home accidents
disease scenarios
liver disease
back pain
bone disease
breast diseases
clubfoot
hip dislocation

contd.

B-7 (*contd.*)

P-3 (contd.)
gallbladder disease
headache
heart diseases
blood pressure (2)
kidney disease
liver disease
motion sickness
muscle disorders
prostate gland enlargement

P-4
backache
birth defect
bone disease
childhood diseases
(digestive) system ailments
gallstones

P-4 (contd.)
food poisoning
scalp problems
hay fever
headache
kidney disease
motion sickness
prostate disorders
weight problems

P-5
blood pressure
collagen diseases
vitamin deficiencies
skin diseases
insect pests
family medicine chest

---

[a] The compound nouns in the above list include single words (e.g. headache, gallstones), as well as double and triple word types.
[b] Bracketed words indicate syntactic context.
[c] Bracketed numbers indicate frequency of occurrence.

B-8
Selected Headings: Prepositional Phrases (Table 45, Graph 45)

The 'List'
(diseases)[a] of the blood . . .
(diseases) of the nervous system . . .
(diseases) of the circulatory system
(diseases) of the respiratory system
(diseases) of the digestive system
(diseases) of the genitourinary system
(complications) of pregnancy . . .
(diseases) of the skin . . .
(diseases) of the musculoskeletal system . . .

contd.

B-8 (*contd.*)

T-1
(approach) to disease
(approach) to clinical medicine
(diseases) of the organ systems
(disorders) of the heart
(disorders) of the vascular system
(disorders) of the respiratory system
(diseases) of the kidneys . . .
(disorders) of the alimentary tract
(disorders) of the hepatobiliary system
(disorders) of the pancreas
(disorders) of the hematopoietic system
(disorders) of the nervous sytem
(diseases) of the striated muscle
(disorders) of bone . . .
(disorders) of joints . . .
(disorders) of supporting tissue

T-2
(the nature) of medicine
(environmental factors) in disease
(diseases) of the joints
(diseases) of unproved etiology
(disorders) of the nervous system . . .
(diseases) of the digestive system
(diseases) of nutrition
(diseases) of metabolism
(diseases) of the endocrine system
(diseases) of bone
(diseases) with significant systemic manifestations
(normal laboratory values) of clinical importance

T-3
(the approach) to the patient
(disorders) of water . . . metabolism
(disturbances) in renal function
(diseases) of the gastrointestinal tract
(diseases) of the liver
(diseases) with abnormalities/of immunity

contd.

B-8 (*contd.*)

T-3 (*contd.*)
(disorders) of the nervous system
(psychiatry) in medicine
(diseases) of medical management
(special topics) in medicine

P-1
(home care) of the patient
(the lungs and chest) in health and disease
(special concerns) of women
(first aid) for your family

P-2
(how to extend your life) with naturomatic healing/of heart . . . disease
(. . . healing methods) for coughs
(how to cope) with disease/by relieving everyday stress/with . . . healing
(how to relieve . . .) with good body mechanics
(first aid . . .) for bruises
(how to relieve . . . pain) with drugless methods/of naturomatic healing
(how to get . . . relief) from backache
(tested . . . methods) for headache
(how to relieve the . . . misery) of stomach ulcers/with naturomatic healing
(how to care) for your teeth/with naturomatic healing methods
(how to treat . . . skin disorders) with naturomatic healing
(how to relieve fatigue . . .) with massage
(how to reverse . . . aging . . .) with naturomatic healing
(how to . . . ease the strain) of the menopause
(miscellaneous . . . remedies) for a variety/of injuries

P-3
0

P-4
(avoiding ailments) of teeth and gums
(toxemia) of pregnancy

contd.

B-8 (*contd.*)

P-5
(symptoms) of disease
(oxygen) in the body
(inheritance) of disease
(aging . . .) of the body
(diseases) of connective tissue
(loss . . .) of weight
(disorders) of bones
(effects) of physical forces/on the body
(the inhaling) of dangerous substances
(the care) of the feet

---

[a] Bracketed words indicate syntactic context.

B-9
Selected Headings: Adverbial Clauses Containing an Infinitive (Table 46, Graph 46)

The 'List'	P-1	P-3
0	0	0
T-1	P-2	P-4
0	How to Extend . . .	0
	How to Cope . . .	
T-2	How to Relieve . . . (4)[a]	P-5
0	How to Get . . .	0
	How to Care for . . .	
T-3	How to Treat . . .	
0	How to Reverse	
	How to Boost . . .	

---

[a] Bracketed numbers indicate frequency of occurrence.

B-10 (a)
Selected Headings: Type One Terms which Name Aberrant States, or which Name Indicators of Aberrant States: Standard vs Nonstandard (Table 47, Graph 47)

The 'List'[a]	T-3	P-3
diseases	diseases (10)	diseases (15)
disorders	disorders (2)	disorders (2)
complications	disturbances	conditions
anomalies	abnormalities	problems (4)
symptoms	problems	pain
signs	emergencies	accidents
injuries		syndrome
poisoning	P-1	
manifestations	diseases (2)	P-4
disturbances	disorders (3)	diseases (6)
abnormalities	illness	disorders (3)
		poisoning
T-1	P-2	problems (2)
diseases (4)[b]	diseases (2)	defects
disorders (16)	disorders	ailments (2)
manifestations	injuries (2)	sickness
	ailments (2)	
T-2	troubles	P-5
diseases (18)	misery	diseases (6)
disorders (2)	pains (4)	disorders (2)
manifestations	aches	symptoms (2)
		poisoning
		disturbances
		complaints
		deficiencies
		breakdown

[a] The lexical items in the 'List' will be assumed to constitute *standard* terms for aberrant states, Type One. Other such terms not appearing in the 'List' will be called *nonstandard* terms for aberrant states, Type One.
[b] Bracketed numbers indicate frequency of occurrence.

B-10 (b)
Distribution of Type One Terms in Selected Headings: 'Standard' vs 'Nonstandard' Terms

'Standard' terms[a]	T-1	T-2	T-3	Total	%[b]	P-1	P-2	P-3	P-4	P-5	Total	%[b]
disease(s)	4	18	10	32		2	2	15	6	6	31	
disorder(s)	16	2	2	20		3	1	1	3	2	10	
complication(s)	—	—	—	—		—	—	—	—	—	—	
anomalies	—	—	—	—		—	—	—	—	—	—	
condition(s)	—	—	—	—		—	—	1	—	—	1	
symptom(s)	—	—	—	—		—	—	—	—	2	2	
sign(s)	—	—	—	—		—	—	—	—	—	—	
injury	—	—	—	—		—	2	—	—	—	2	
poisoning	—	—	—	—		—	—	—	1	1	2	
manifestation(s)	1	1	—	2		—	—	—	1	—	1	
disturbance(s)	—	—	1	1		—	—	—	—	1	1	
abnormalities	—	—	1	1		—	—	—	—	—	—	
Total no. of Standard Terms	21	21	14	56	97	5	5	17	10	12	49	65

contd.

B-10 (b) *(contd.)*

'Nonstandard' terms[c]	T-1	T-2	T-3	Total	%[b]	P-1	P-2	P-3	P-4	P-5	Total	%[b]
problem(s)	–	–	1	1		–	–	4	2	–	6	
defect(s)	–	–	–	–		–	–	–	1	–	1	
ailment(s)	–	–	–	–		–	2	–	2	–	4	
illness(es)	–	–	–	–		1	–	–	–	–	1	
complaint(s)	–	–	–	–		–	–	–	–	1	1	
deficiencies	–	–	–	–		–	–	–	–	1	1	
trouble(s)	–	–	–	–		–	1	–	–	–	1	
misery	–	–	–	–		–	1	–	–	–	1	
pain(s)	–	–	–	–		–	4	1	–	–	5	
ache(s)	–	–	–	–		–	1	–	–	–	1	
sickness	–	–	–	–		–	–	–	1	–	1	
accidents	–	–	–	–		–	–	1	–	–	1	
emergencies	–	–	1	1		–	–	–	–	–	–	
breakdown	–	–	–	–		–	–	–	–	1	1	
syndrome	–	–	–	–		–	–	1	–	–	1	
Total no. of Nonstandard Terms	0	0	2	2	3	1	9	7	6	3	26	35

[a] The 12 Type One terms appearing in this list are identified as standard by reason of the fact that they all occur in the 'List of Three-digit Categories'.

[b] Based on the total number of terms for aberrant states, Type One, in each group.

[c] The 15 Type One terms appearing in list do not appear in the 'List of Three-digit Categories', hence are called 'non-standard'.

B-10 (c)
Type One Terms: Class T,[a] Class P,[b] and Class T ∩ P[c]

Class T Terms	Class P Terms	Class T ∩ P Terms
manifestations[d]	conditions[a]	diseases[d]
abnormalities[d]	symptoms[d]	disorders[d]
emergencies	injuries[d]	disturbances[d]
	poisoning[d]	problems
	defects	
	ailments	
	illnesses	
	complaints	
	deficiencies	
	troubles	
	misery	
	pains	
	aches	
	sickness	
	accidents	
	breakdown	
	syndrome	

[a] Exclusive to (Selected Headings of) textbooks.
[b] Exclusive to (Selected Headings of) popular books.
[c] Common to (Selected Headings of) both textbooks and popular books.
[d] 'Standard' terms (i.e. those appearing on the 'List of Three-digit Categories').

B-11
Selected Headings: Type Two Terms which Name Aberrant States, or which Name Indicators of Aberrant States (Table 48, Graph 48)

The 'List'	P-1
neoplasms	cancer
	hypersensitivity
T-1	allergies
0	arthritis
	rheumatism
T-2	
rheumatoid arthritis	P-2
	stress
T-3	tension
0	coughs

contd.

B-11 (*contd.*)

P-2 (*contd.*)
colds
sore throat
headache
constipation
hemorrhoids
stomach ulcers
colitis
bruises
strains
sprains
backache
arthritis
fatigue

P-3
Addison's disease
allergy
amebiasis
amebic dysentery
amebic liver disease
anemias
appendicitis
asthma
low back pain
bronchitis
emphysema
brucellosis
undulant fever
bursitis
cancer
cerebral palsy
clubfoot
congenital hip dislocation
common cold
Cushing's syndrome
adrenal cortical hyperfunction
diabetes
dizziness
Meniere's disease
epilepsy
gonorrhea

venereal diseases
headache
migraine
hemophilia
hemorrhoids
hernia
high blood pressure
hypertension
Hodgkin's disease
leprosy
Hansen's disease
leukemia
low blood pressure
malaria
menstrual disorders
fibroids
infectious mononucleosis
motion sickness
multiple sclerosis
myasthenia gravis
narcolepsy
Parkinson's disease
pneumonias
poliomyelitis
prostate gland enlargement
psoriasis
purpura
sarcoidosis
Boeck's sarcoid
schizophrenia
sciatica
stroke
suicide
syphilis
tuberculosis
ulcer (stomach & duodenoum)
ulcer (peptic)
ulcerative colitis
varicose veins

P-4
allergy

contd.

B-11 *(contd.)*

P-4 (contd.)
anemia
arthritis
asthma
backache
bad breath
bedwetting
bronchitis
cancer
celiac disease
colds
constipation
diabetes
diarrhea
diverticulitis
emphysema
epilepsy
food poisoning
gallstones
goiter
hay fever
headache
hemorrhoids
hernia

insomnia
miscarriage
mononucleosis
motion sickness
multiple sclerosis
muscular dystrophy
Parkinson's disease
rabies
shingles
sinusitis
tetany
tonsillitis
toxemia of pregnancy
tuberculosis
ulcers
varicose veins
venereal diseases

P-5
fevers
infections
cancer
stress
venereal diseases

B-12
Selected Headings: Terms Belonging to the Domain of Treatment or Care of the Human Organism (Table 49, Graph 49)

The 'List'
0

T-1
clinical pharmacology

T-2
0

T-3
(diseases of medical)[a] management

P-1
(home) care
(child) care
(the teeth and their) care
(your) operation
drug (use)
(first) aid

P-2
healing (10)[b]
relieving

contd.

B-12 (*contd.*)

P-2 (contd.)
relieve (4)
good body mechanics
(foot) care
(first) aid
(drugless) methods
relief
care (for your teeth)
treat (skin disorders)
rejuvenate (your body)
massage
tonics
ease (the strain of)
remedies

(weight) control
(body) care
(mental) care
(family preventive) care
(medical) reinforcements
help (for emotional problems)
(other) helps
counseling

P-4
0

P-5
care (of the feet)
(first) aid

P-3
(preventive) therapy

---

[a] Bracketed words indicate syntactic context.
[b] Bracketed numbers indicate frequency of occurrence.

B-13
Selected Headings: The Terms 'Health', 'Prevention', and Their Variants
(Table 50, Graph 50)

The 'List'	*P-2*
0	0

T-1
0

T-2
0

T-3
0

P-1
health (and disease)[a]

P-3
(accidents and their) prevention
preventive (medicine) (2)[b]
preventive (therapy)
preventive (body care)
preventive (mental care)
preventive (psychiatry)
(family) preventive (care)
(building general) health
(your) health
healthy (adjustment in marriage)
healthy (parenthood)

contd.

B-13 (*contd.*)

P-4	*P-5*
avoiding (ailments)	(mental) health

---

[a] Bracketed words indicate syntactic context.
[b] Bracketed numbers indicate frequency of occurrence.

B-14
Selected Headings: The Term 'Body' (Table 51, Graph 51)

The 'List'	*P-3*
0	(strength of the human) body
	body (care)
T-1	body (defences)
0	(mind,) body, (mind)
T-2	*P-4*
0	0
T-3	*P-5*
0	(oxygen in the) body
	(breakdown of the) body
P-1	(effects of physical forces on the)
0	body
P-2	
body (mechanics)	

B-15 (a)
Selected Headings: The Term 'System' or Its Variants (Table 52, Graph 52)

The 'List'[a]	(respiratory) system
(nervous) system	(vascular) system
(circulatory) system	(organ) system
(respiratory) system	(hepatobiliary) system
(digestive) system	(hematopoietic) system
(genitourinary) system	
(musculoskeletal) system	*T-2*
	(nervous) system
T-1	(digestive) system
(nervous) system	(organ) system

contd.

B-15 (a) (*contd.*)

T-2 (contd.)
(endocrine) system
systemic (manifestations)

T-3
(nervous) system

P-1
(nervous) system
(circulatory) system
(digestive) system

P-2
0

P-3
(nervous) system
(circulatory) system
(respiratory) system
(digestive) system
(genitourinary) system
(skeletal) system

P-4
(digestive) system

P-5
0

---

[a] The six bracketed words placed under the 'List' will be taken as 'standard' terms for kinds of systems. The relative distribution of 'standard' vs 'non-standard' terms for kinds of systems will be indicated in the display on the following page.

B-15 (b)
Distribution of Terms Indicating Kinds of Systems: 'Standard' vs 'Non-standard' Terms

	T-1	T-2	T-3	Total	P-1	P-2	P-3	P-4	P-5	Total
Total no. of different kinds of systems cited	6	4	1	11	3	0	6	1	0	10

	T-1	T-2	T-3	Total	%[a]	P-1	P-2	P-3	P-4	P-5	Total	%[a]
'Standard' Terms												
nervous	1	1	1	3		1	–	1	–	–	2	
circulatory	–	–	–	0		1	–	1	–	–	2	
respiratory	1	–	–	1		–	–	1	–	–	1	
digestive	–	1	–	1		1	–	1	1	–	3	
genitourinary	–	–	–	0		–	–	1	–	–	1	
musculoskeletal	–	–	–	0		–	–	–	–	–	0	
Total	2	2	1	5	45	3	0	5	1	0	9	90

contd.

B-15 (b) *(contd.)*

	T-1	T-2	T-3	Total	%[a]	P-1	P-2	P-3	P-4	P-5	Total	%[a]
'Nonstandard'												
Terms												
skeletal	—	—	—	0		—	—	1	—	—	1	
vascular	1	—	—	1		—	—	—	—	—	0	
organ	1	1	—	2		—	—	—	—	—	0	
hepatobiliary	1	—	—	1		—	—	––	—	—	0	
hematopoietic	1	—	—	1		—	—	—	—	—	0	
endocrine	—	1	—	1		—	—	—	—	—	0	
Total	4	2	0	6	55	0	0	1	0	0	1	10

[a] Based on total number of 'standard' and 'non-standard' terms for each group.

B-15 (c)

All Terms Indicating Kinds of Systems Grouped into Three Classes: T,[a] P,[b] and $T \cap P$[c]

Class T Terms	Class P Terms	Class T ∩ P Terms
vascular	circulatory[d]	nervous[d]
organ	genitourinary[d]	respiratory[d]
hepatobiliary	skeletal	digestive[d]
hematopoietic		
endocrine		

[a] Exclusive to (Selected Headings of) textbooks.
[b] Exclusive to (Selected Headings of) popular books.
[c] Common to (Selected Headings of) both textbooks and popular books.
[d] Standard terms (i.e. those appearing in the 'List of Three-digit Categories').

B-16

Selected Headings: Nouns which Name Specific Anatomical Structures[a] of the Human Organism: 'Covert' vs 'Overt' Structures[b] (Table 53, Graph 53)

'Covert' Structures	'Overt' Structures
The 'List'	*The 'List'*
blood-forming organs	sense organs

contd.

B-16 (*contd.*)

'Covert' Structures	'Overt' Structures
The 'List' (*contd.*)	*The 'List'* (*contd.*)
subcutaneous tissue	skin
connective tissue	
T-1	*T-1*
heart	0
kidneys	
urinary tract	
alimentary tract	
pancreas	
striated muscle	
bone	
joints	
connective tissue	
supportive tissue	
T-2	*T-2*
connective tissue	0
joints	
bone	
T-3	*T-3*
gastrointestinal tract	0
liver	
P-1	*P-1*
heart	skin
blood-forming organs	chest
lungs	teeth
kidneys	eyes
genitourinary tract	ears
endocrine glands	nose
bones	throat
muscles	
P-2	*P-2*
heart	throat
blood vessel (disease)[c]	foot
muscle	neck
stomach	arm

contd.

B-16 (*contd.*)

'Covert' Structures	'Overt' Structures
P-2 (*contd.*)	*P-2* (*contd.*)
bones	shoulder
joints	leg
	teeth
	gums
	skin
P-3	*P-3*
muscle(s) (2)[d]	skin
brain	hair
endocrine glands	nails
liver (2)	sense organs
bone	teeth
gallbladder (disease)	feet
heart	back
kidney	breast
prostate gland	hip
sinuses	
stomach	
duodenum	
veins	
P-4	*P-4*
appendix	ears
bone	eyes
heart	feet
kidney	hair
liver	scalp
prostate	skin
veins	teeth
	gums
P-5	*P-5*
heart	skin
kidneys	eyes
connective tissue	nose
endocrine glands	throat
bones	ear
	feet

contd.

B-16 (*contd.*)

[a] That is, tissues, organs, glands, or other 'parts'.
[b] The distinction between 'covert' and 'overt' anatomical structures has been made on the basis of the fact that the former are, relatively speaking, both hidden to the eye and unpalpable by the untrained hand, whereas the latter are readily visible and/or accessible to touch.
[c] Bracketed words indicate syntactic context.
[d] Bracketed numbers indicate frequency of occurrence. . . . .

B-17
Selected Heading: Terms Belonging to the Domains of Psychiatry, Neurology, or Behavioral Psychology (Table 54, Graph 54)

The 'List'
mental (disorders)[a]
nervous (system)

T-1
nervous (system)
psychiatric (disorders)

T-2
nervous (system)
(disorders of) behavior

T-3
nervous (system)
psychiatry
alcoholism

P-1
emotional (illness)
mental
nervous (system)

P-2
aches
pains
stress
tension
fatigue

P-3
sleep
relaxation
smoking
drinking
brain
nervous (system)
mental (care)
mental (problems)
mind (2)[b]
emotional (problems)
psychiatry
pain
cerebral palsy
dizziness
epilepsy
headache
migraine
myasthenia gravis
narcolepsy
Parkinson's disease
poliomyelitis
schizophrenia
sciatica
senility
stroke
suicide

contd.

B-17 (*contd.*)

P-4
alcoholism
bedwetting
emotional (disorders)
nervous (disorders)
epilepsy
headache
insomnia
motion sickness

P-4 (*contd.*)
multiple sclerosis
Parkinson's disease

P-5
emotional (development)
mental
stress
mental (health)

---

[a] Bracketed words indicate syntactic context.
[b] Bracketed numbers indicate frequency of occurrence.

B-18
Selected Headings: Terms which Name Certain Sexual, Social, and Developmental States or Roles of the Human Organism (Table 55, Graph 55)

The 'List'
pregnancy
childbirth
puerperium
perinatal (period)[a]

T-1
0

T-2
0

T-3
adolescent (medicine)

P-1
pregnancy
childbirth
infant
child
home
family
women

P-2
aging
(how to remain) younger
sex (life)
menopause
male
climacteric

P-3
sexual (adjustment)
family
marriage (3)[b]
home
work
parenthood
aging
venereal diseases
menopause
menstrual (disorders)
senility

P-4
birth (defects)
miscarriage

contd.

B-18 (*contd.*)

P-4 (contd.)	*P-5*
venereal diseases	aging
childhood (diseases)	breakdown (of the body)
sexual (disorders)	venereal diseases
(toxemia of) pregnancy	family (medicine chest)
	vacation
	(emotional) development

[a] Bracketed words indicate syntactic context.
[b] Bracketed numbers indicate frequency of occurrence.

B-19
Selected Headings: Terms which Name So-called 'Natural' Approaches to the Maintenance of Health (Table 56, Graph 56)

The 'List'	*P-2*
nutritional (diseases)[a]	naturomatic (10)[b] (healing)
	naturomatic (remedies)
T-1	naturomatic (tonics)
nutritional (disorders)	nature's (way)
	drugless (methods)
T-2	massage
(diseases of) nutrition	
	P-3
T-3	foods (you eat)
0	weight (control)
	physical activity
P-1	sleep
weight (problems)	relaxation
	P-4
	weight (problems)
	P-5
	(loss and gain of) weight
	vitamin (deficiencies)
	exercise

[a] Bracketed words indicate syntactic context.
[b] Bracketed numbers indicate frequency of occurrence.

3.   THE PARATEXT

a.   *Its composition*

The Paratext is that segment of a book which includes all portions except the Text and the Table of Contents. Upon inspection, Paratextual components (some of which precede the Table of Contents and others of which follow the Text) reveal a number of interesting features, particularly with respect to the present study.

b.   *Its purpose*

The various elements of the Paratext fulfil a number of different functions, for example:

(i)   The Index facilitates rapid retrieval of information from the Text by presenting an alphabeticized list of important substantive terms (including proper nouns) followed by an indication of the locations of the various contexts in which such terms have been elaborated.[28]

(ii)   Data pertaining to the publishing history of the book (editions, copyrights, translations, etc.) establish the book's legal and international status.

(iii)   Acknowledgements and dedications reveal the social and professional affiliations of the author or editor.

(iv)   Introductory discourse (i.e. prefaces, introductions, forewords, etc.) indicate the goals and ideological biases of the author or editor.

c.   *Objectives of investigation*

(i)   To determine which Paratextual components are characteristically present or absent in textbooks as compared to popular books (see Table 58 which follows).

(ii)   To determine (on the basis of statements made in the introductory discourse) in which respects the editorial stances of textbooks differ from the editorial stances of popular books.

Table 58.   *Distribution of Paratextual components in textbooks vs popular Books*

Name of Component	T-1	T-2	T-3	P-1	P-2	P-3	P-4	P-5
A. *Introductory discourse:*								
1. Foreword	○	○	●	●	●	○	○	○
2. Introduction	○	○	○	○	●	○	●	●
3. Preface	●	●	●	○	○	○	○-	●
B. *Other components*								
1. Acknowledgement [b]	○	○	○	○	○	●	○	○
2. Appendix	●	○	●	●	○	○	○	●
3. Dedication	●	●	●	○	●	●	○	●
4. Glossary of Medical Terms	○	○	○	●	○	○	○	●
5. Index	●	●	●	●	●	●	●	●
6. List of Contributors and Their Credentials	●	●	●	●	○	○	○	○
7. List of Previous Editors	●	○	○	○	○	○	○	○
8. List of Other Books by Author or Editor	○	○	○	●	●	○	○	○
9. Photograph of Author or Editor	○	○	○	●	○	○	○	○
10. Warning Concerning Drug Administration and Therapy	●	○	●	○	○	○	○	○
11. Information Concerning Number of Recent Translations	●	●	○	○	○	○	○	○
Total	8	5	8	7	4	3	2	6

● = component is present in the Paratext.
○ = component is absent in the Paratext.
[a] T-3 has two Prefaces.
[b] In textbooks, acknowledgements are located in the Preface.

Objective (ii) (see above) has been approached by examining introductory discourse in terms of expressed or implied attitudes concerning (continued on p. 189):

Graph 58.   *Distribution of Paratextual components in textbooks vs popular books*

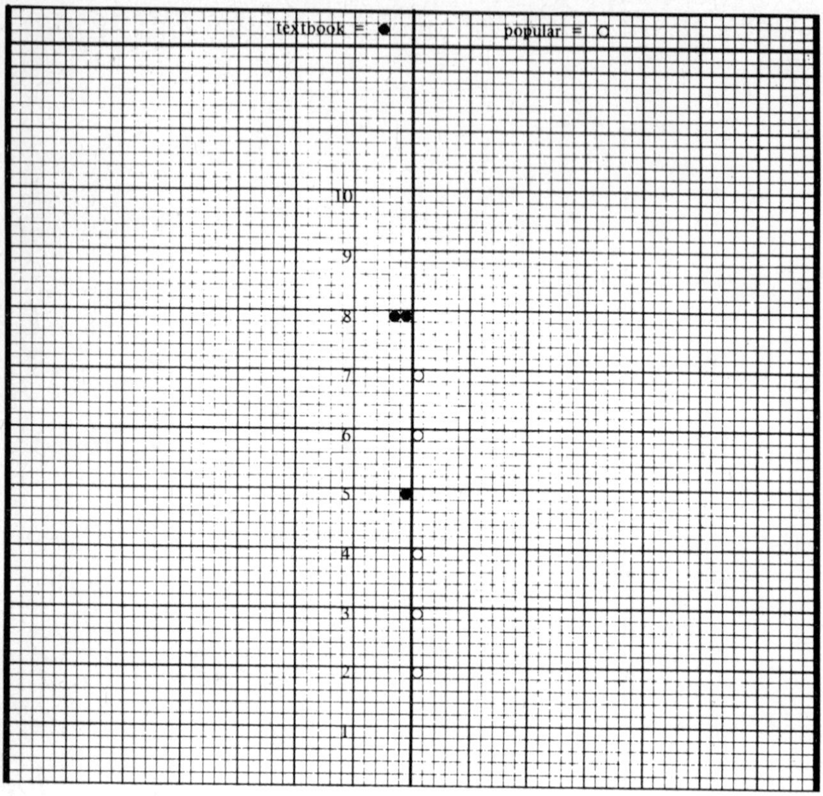

[a]   the perceived function of the book;
[b]   physicians;
[c]   the readers.

On the basis of statements taken from the introductory discourse of each of the eight selected books,[29] the writer will now attempt to indicate the editorial stance of each book. In each case, the academic status of the writer(s) *of the discourse* will first be indicated.

Comparison of editorial stance: textbook vs popular

Editorial stance of T-1[30]

Status of writers (5):   *M.D.:* X   *Other:*

[a]   *The perceived function of the book.* (i) To teach 'a logical approach to the consideration of the patient's complaints' (C-1 (a), lines 71-72), and (ii) to encourage a 'critical' attitude in the readers, both of the above in the service of educating the intended 'consumer' of the book.

With respect to (i) above, the editors specify that they wish to 'recapitulate the steps in the process of thinking by which a physician reaches a diagnosis' (C-1 (a), lines 20-22) 'within the clinical setting' (C-1 (a), line 54). According to the editors, such 'steps' involve an identification of the 'cardinal manifestations', i.e. the signs and symptoms of disease (C-1 (a), lines 29-30), their 'different causes' (C-1 (a), line 32), the 'syndromes' within which such signs and symptoms occur (C-1 (a), line 57), the various 'disease mechanisms' (C-1 (a), line 59) which may have produced them, including their biochemical and pathophysiological bases (C-1 (a), lines 52-53), following upon which one may then take 'measures to restore the normal physiologic state . . . in a logical, systematic fashion' (C-1 (a), lines 60-62).

With respect to (ii) above, the editors state that '. . . Dr. Wintrobe and his associates . . . sponsored the unique system of critical review of each new chapter by medical students and house staff as well as faculty members, thus giving the editors very helpful insight into the needs and ideas of the "consumer" ' (C-1 (a), lines 109-114).

[b]   *Physicians.* An assumption is made that those physicians involved in the preparation of T-1 are committed to a logical and critical approach towards the teaching of clinical medicine.

[c]   *The Reader.* The probable readers or 'consumers' of T-1 are, by implication, 'medical students . . . house staff . . . (and) faculty members' (C-1 (a), lines 111-112); in short, those who belong to the medical profession. An underlying assumption is that such readers are likely to subscribe to the logical and critical approach emphasized by the editors.

Editorial stance of T-2[31]

Status of writer(s) (2):   *M.D.:* X   *Other:*

[a]   *The perceived function of the book.* The book is described as 'a classical medical text' (C-1 (b), line 77); one, however, which is 'less the repository of established doctrine and more the expression of advanced, ongoing ideas in medicine' (C-1 (b), lines 25-27). The editors claim that 'a major goal in this edition has been to give as much information as practical about therapy' (C-1 (b), lines 63-64), and they take on as their 'legacy' (C-1 (b), line 38) the task of 'exert[ing] a healing influence on the many thousands of patients they never got to see and a learning influence on the many thousands of students who could not know personally their extraordinary dedication to teaching' (C-1 (b), lines 33-37).

[b]   *Physicians.* The physician-editors typify themselves as dedicated to the traditions established by previous editors: '. . . we gladly accepted (becoming coeditors) with the goal of striving to maintain the high standards set by our predecessors' (C-1 (b), lines 44-45), and 'we view seriously our responsibility as custodians of what has become a classical medical text' (C-1 (b), lines 76-77).

[c]   *The reader.* The intended readers are 'physicians and medical students' (C-1 (b), lines 23 and 28-29) involved in clinical medicine.

Editorial stance of T-3[32]

Status of writer(s) (4):   *M.D.:* X   *Other:*

[a]   *Perceived function of the book.* It is emphasized that T-3 is 'clearly not a revision of Dr. Osler's great book' (C-1 (c), line 27), and that 'the basic theme of this textbook has been the approach to medical practice as exemplified by the staff of a single Department of Medicine . . . (at) Johns Hopkins' (C-1 (c), lines 40-44).

The editors (i) claim that 'It is our purpose to produce a book which is built around the patient rather than the disease' (C-1 (c), lines 73-74), (ii) imply that they will address 'the confusing complexities which arise in the day-to-day investigation and management of clinical problems' (C-1 (c), lines 65-66), and (iii) propose that the physician deal 'systematically' (C-1 (c), line 59) with three basic questions:
'1.   What is the matter with the patient?
2.   What can I do for him?
3.   What will be the outcome?' (C-1 (c), lines 51-53).
Moreover, the editors suggest that T-3 be read in conjunction with other textbooks in order 'to fill the gaps in his knowledge of the subject in hand' (C-1 (c), lines 91-92) for, 'in order to devote more space to the sequential steps which should be taken by the physician seeking the answers to his three basic questions, we have avoided . . . duplication of the type of presentation so successfully employed in texts already available' (C-1 (c), lines 84-89). Hence the book is intended to 'complement the existent encyclopedic texts' (C-1 (c), lines 22-23).

[b]   *Physicians.* It is claimed that the physician-editors are committed to 'the preservation of a heritage of clinical excellence' (C-1 (c), lines 29-30). Moreover, they endorse both the value of 'constructive criticism' (C-1 (c), line 46) as well as the value of self-criticism (as is evident from the inclusion of Section Seventeen of T-3: 'Diseases of Medical Management').

Editorial stance of P-1[33]

Status of writer (1):   *M.D.:*   *Other:* X

[a]   *The perceived function of the book.* The book purports (i) to demystify medical concepts and medical language, (ii) to inform the reader about health problems, prevention, etc., and (iii) to fill in a 'communications gap' between the doctor and the patient.
With respect to (i) above, the editor claims that 'We explain unfamiliar technical terms; none have we avoided, as many "doctor's words" are now part of the common language' (C-1 (d), lines 22-24), that the book's 'illustrations illuminate the wondrous mechanisms of the body . . .' (C-1 (d), lines 20-21) and that the book's contributors are able 'to dispel misconceptions' (C-1 (d), line 31).
With respect to (ii) above, the editor states that the book provides

'authoritative information about health problems . . . as well as practical matters of appropriate home care, prevention of disease, maintenance of health, and recognition of illness . . .' (C-1 (d), lines 13-18).

With respect to (iii) above, the editor states that the book has been designed 'to supplement the counsel of one's own personal physician' (C-1 (d), lines 5-6) and that 'If this book helps to make you a more understanding patient, then it's surely the indispensable complement to an understanding doctor' (C-1 (d), lines 34-36).

[b]   *Physicians.* The Foreword of P-1 reveals an ambiguous attitude towards the physician. On the one hand, the medical contributors to the book are respectfully typified as 'a corps of medical men which includes . . . America's most distinguished specialists and authorities' (C-1 (d), lines 2-4), and as 'eminent physicians' (C-1 (d), line 25); also (with respect to other physicians), it is stated that '. . . one's own personal physician . . . [is] alone competent to diagnose and treat conditions in individual patients' (C-1 (d), lines 5-7), and that [he] 'has the great resources of modern medicine at his and your disposal' (C-1 (d), lines 18-20). However, physicians in general are typified as being busy, thus (by innuendo), negligent in communicating satisfactorily with the patient: '. . . doctors can rarely take the time to explain [things] to us' (C-1 (d), lines 10-11) and 'We invited each contributor to discuss his topic as if he . . . [had] all the time in the world to give counsel and to dispel misconceptions' (C-1 (d), lines 28-31).

[c]   *The reader.* The reader is typified as 'intelligent' (C-1 (d), lines 8 and 30), as 'concerned' (C-1 (d), line 30), as capable of 'understanding' (C-1 (d), line 35), and as having a 'family and personal life' (C-1 (d), line 15).

Finally, that the contributors to the book include 'eminent physicians', is interpreted by the writer as an endorsement by significant members of the medical profession (C-1 (d), lines 25-28).

Editorial stance of P-2[34]

Status of writer(s) (2). P-2 has two samples of introductory discourse, one entitled 'Foreword By A Doctor of Medicine', and the other, 'What This Book Can Do For You', by a chiropractor (the book's author).

[a]   *Perceived function of the book.* The book is claimed to be an 'easy-to-read' health guide (C-1 (e), line 75) that (i) is economical to the reader and (ii) endorses 'Naturomatic Healing Methods'.

With respect to (i) above, the writer claims that 'regular use of this book will cut down your health expenses . . .' (C-1 (e), lines 60-61).

With respect to (ii) above, Naturomatic Healing is defined as 'the whole system of natural[35] healing which . . . seems to work automatically to help your body heal itself, and restore its natural health balance' (C-1 (e), lines 102-104). The writer provides the reader access to this 'system' through the presentation of 'home remedies' which combine 'healing science with "folk medicine" and "health secrets" in a self-help program . . .' (C-1 (e), lines 80-82).

[b] *Physicians.* The physician is typified as (i) consistently busy, hence, by implication, negligent in certain of his responsibilities, and (ii) expensive.

With respect to (i) above, the writer states that 'unfortunately, few doctors have the time to tell their patients how to help themselves' (C-1 (e), lines 38-39). Also, because doctors are 'so overworked', 'only "serious" disorders receive adequate attention in the average doctor's office. The truth is, however, that many "minor" disorders can develop into serious disease when they are neglected' (C-1 (e), lines 40-43). Finally, the reader is advised: 'You don't have to run to an overworked doctor's office every time you have a muscle spasm, a cold, or a headache' (C-1 (e), lines 64-66).

With respect to (ii) above, the writer claims that 'the average family spends several hundred dollars and upwards each year on medical bills' (C-1 (e), lines 34-35), and advises the reader that 'you can care for many of your ailments as effectively as the most expensive specialist' (C-1 (e), lines 63-64).

[c] *The reader.* The reader is treated as one who (i) is sympathetic to the value of thrift, (ii) is sympathetic to the value of self-sufficiency, (iii) will be satisfied with simple explanations concerning natural methods of promoting health and longevity, and alleviating minor or chronic disorders, (iv) may have become disenchanted with results obtained through conventional medicine, and (v) is living at home within a family environment.

With respect to (i) above, the writer emphasizes that 'regular use of this book will cut down your health expenses . . .' (C-1 (e), lines 60-61), and that 'for less than the price of one office call, you can acquire more health guidance from this book than a doctor could give you in a hundred office calls . . .' (C-1 (e), lines 57-59).

With respect to (ii) above, the writer states that 'your body has a remarkable ability to heal itself when it is helped along by natural healing methods' (C-1 (e), lines 51-53). Also, the book is intended for 'people who want to help themselves' (C-1 (e), lines 12-13), with the writer emphasizing that 'you are personally responsible for your health and the care of your body' (C-1 (e), lines 17-18), and that 'you alone must make the final judgment of the effectiveness of remedies and measures that affect your health' (C-1 (e), lines 22-24).

With respect to (iii) above, the writer promises 'a handy and easy-to-read guide to reliable and effective natural remedies . . .' (C-1 (e), lines 75-76). Such 'drugless remedies' (C-1 (e), line 29) can 'improv[e] . . . your health and prolong [. . .] life' (C-1 (e), lines 73-74). Also, 'there are millions of people who are suffering from minor and chronic ailments that would respond immediately to properly applied natural remedies' (C-1 (e), lines 47-49).

With respect to (iv) above, the writer claims that 'a new spinal manipulation technique . . . can be used safely at home by anyone, (and) will do wonders in relieving aches and pains that do not respond to conventional treatment methods' (C-1 (e), lines 88-91). Also, the writer claims that he can bring to the reader 'many new and effective treatment methods that have been designed to produce rapid and lasting results' (C-1 (e), lines 92-94).

With respect to (v) above, the writer states that 'suffering could be relieved at home' (C-1 (e), line 49), and suggests that such natural remedies as are outlined in the book 'can be used by every member of your family' (C-1 (e), line 76-77).

In summary, P-2 represents an interesting blend of all three 'traditions' of domestic literature indicated in Part One, Section II: 4 — the 'Buchan tradition' (because it purports to enlighten the reader), the 'Wesley tradition' (because of its attitude towards doctors), and the 'recipe tradition' (both because of its promise of 'health secrets' as well as the recipe format of certain portions of its contents).

Editorial stance of P-3[36]

Status of writer(s) (5):   M.D.:   Other: X

[a]   *Perceived function of the book.* According to the writers, 'Our aim in writing this book . . . (is) to provide . . . a detailed guide to the concepts and practices of preventive medicine—how the physician uses them and how the individual can apply them' (C-1 (f), lines 94-97).

Towards this end, the writers describe three stages of prevention: primary, which is to 'prevent disease from happening' (C-1 (f), line 51), 'secondary', which is to prevent existent disease from progressing (C-1 (f), line 53), and 'tertiary', to 'hold [. . .] in check . . . even far-advanced disease so that radical measures, such as organ substitution when applicable, may be used' (C-1 (f), lines 55-57).

In short, the basic maxim of the book is that 'treatment never equals prevention . . . [for] treatment does not always work; even when it does, it may eliminate the disease but not the damage already done. It is prevention that must be counted upon to make the big inroads against both death and disability' (C-1 (f), lines 12-17).

[b] *Physicians.* According to the writers, the 'preventively-minded physician' (C-1 (f), line 168) is:

(i) cognizant of data pertaining to the patient's medical history and socioeconomic status (C-1 (f), lines 170-174);

(ii) involved in a periodic, long-term relationship with the patient (C-1 (f), lines 175-176);

(iii) attuned to the patient's mental and emotional states (C-1 (f), lines 183-184), the patient's living habits (C-1 (f), line 186) and the possible effects of both of the above upon the patient's health (C-1 (f), line 187);

(iv) 'prepared to intervene' at the first signs of approaching disease (C-1 (f), lines 192-193).

With respect to (iv) above, the modern physician is described as having powerful predictive skills: 'Medicine [has begun] to penetrate the mysteries of psychic disease . . .' (C-1 (f), line 110) and 'medicine has been developing a kind of scientific crystal ball that promises to make far greater inroads on disease, that can be rubbed to see the portents for the individual patient . . .' (C-1 (f), lines 119-122).

On the basis of this predictive knowledge, the writers assign the physicians considerable control in the 'government' of the patient's state or condition:

As medicine has been practiced generally to now, it has been the patient who, in effect, has turned up after making a self-diagnosis. It has been the patient who has decided, 'I think I am or may be sick or becoming sick', and then has sought help.

Now it will be the preventively minded physician who increasingly will be able to tell the patient, 'You are about to become sick and we are going to take a few measures in advance so you won't actually develop the sickness (C-1 (f), lines 199-212).

Finally, according to the writers, the traditionally-minded physician must share the credit for advances in health with 'the sanitary engineer, the agriculturist, the public health officer, the pediatrician, and the family physician practicing preventive medicine' (C-1 (f), lines 18-21).

[c] *The reader.* The reader is identified as (i) American, (ii) altruistic, (iii)

unhealthy, (iv) highly prone to getting sick, particularly if he belongs to certain groups definable by age, sex, family history, race, and occupation, (v) receptive to arguments based on statistical data, and (vi) concerned about aging.

With respect to (i) and (ii) above, the writers state that 'We Americans, a warmhearted people, like to rally round to "help the handicapped" . . .' (C-1 (f), lines 62-63).

With respect to (iii) above, the writers declare that 'many of us . . . belong among the handicapped' (C-1 (f), lines 64-66), that 'If not outrightly sick, we are never fully healthy' (C-1 (f), line 67), and that advertising on television is an indication of our need for remedies for 'tired feelings, stomach upsets, heartburn, acid indigestion, insomnia, tension, a multitude of aches and pains' (C-1 (f), lines 73-75).

With respect to (iv) above, the writers point out that 'in the Korean War, autopsies of young American soldiers revealed that in 54 percent of these youths . . . coronary heart disease was already starting. No longer could the disease be considered degenerative, a part of aging' (C-1 (f), lines 157-161). Moreover, with respect to proneness, the writers point out the high risk of breast cancer in women whose female relatives have also had the disease, of stomach cancer amongst the Japanese, of nose and throat cancer among the Chinese and Malaysians, of stomach and cervical cancer amongst American workers and their wives, and of bladder cancer amongst aniline dye workers (C-1 (f), lines 129-153).

With respect to (v) above, see C-1 (f), lines 129-134 and line 158.

With respect to (vi) above, see C-1 (f), lines 78-82.

Editorial stance of P-4[37]

Status of writer (1):   *M.D.:*   *Other:* X

[a]   *Perceived function of the book.* This 'useful, understandable' book (C-1 (g), lines 32-33) which is described as 'a blueprint for better, more healthful living' (C-1 (g), line 44) promulgates the following values: (i) healthful, natural living, (ii) patient education, (iii) prevention, and (iv) medical science.

With respect to (i) above, the writer claims that 'health comes from the way people live, not from doctors and hospitals' (C-1 (g), lines 42-43), and that 'natural is best' (C-1 (g), line 35), i.e. 'when there is solid scientific evidence that drugless, non-surgical treatments have proven effective, they are emphasized' (C-1 (g), lines 35-37).

With respect to (ii) above, the writer states that 'the informed patient understands, more readily, the symptoms of his illness and the aims of his treatment . . . and is prepared to ask the doctor the right questions and volunteer important information that can help in his treatment' (C-1 (g), lines 23-27).

With respect to (iii) above, the writer states that 'the person who identifies . . . threats (to the body) and tries to avoid them is taking the most important steps there are in battling disease' (C-1 (g), lines 30-32).

With respect to (iv) above, the writer claims that 'each disease section has been carefully researched for the latest information and all medical and scientific conclusions are based on reports from the most respected of the world's medical and scientific journals' (C-1 (g), lines 17-20).

[b] *Physicians.* Firstly, the doctor is identified with 'the world of science as it relates to health' (C-1 (g), line 1), whose 'miraculous advances' (C-1 (g), line 41), some of which the writer lists (C-1 (g), lines 3-6) are clearly acknowledged. Secondly, the doctor is presented as the ultimate authority on 'serious illness (with respect to which) no book, however thorough it might be, can take the place of a consultation with a physician' (C-1 (g), lines 21-23). Finally, however, the doctor is disqualified as a source of health, for, 'as a rule, health [does not come] . . . from doctors and hospitals' (C-1 (g), lines 42-43).

[c] *The reader.* The reader is assumed to be sympathetic to the values of (i) self-sufficiency and (ii) prevention.

With respect to (i) above, the writer emphasizes that 'every person is responsible for his own health' (C-1 (g), line 28).

With respect to (ii) above, the writer emphasizes the value of avoiding disease (C-1 (g), lines 30-32).

Editorial stance of P-5[38]

Status of writer (1):   *M.D.:* X   *Other:*

[a] *The perceived function of the book.* The function of the book is perceived as that of ultimately facilitating the doctor's task in dealing with the patient. 'This book, it is hoped, will give the reader a better understanding of his own medical troubles and thereby make him a better patient for his doctor' (C-1 (h), lines 26-28).

[b] *Physicians.* The doctor is identified as belonging to a tradition of 'medical science' (C-1 (h), line 1), and is described as one who is competent in

interpreting a patient's 'symptom or disturbance' (C-1 (h), lines 15-16) both in light of technological procedures, such as 'X-ray, or a variety of laboratory examinations' (C-1 (h), lines 22-23) as well as in light of 'a record of all his previous diseases, and a most intimate search into the condition for which he consults a physician' (C-1 (h), lines 23-25).

[c]   *The reader.* The reader is addressed as one who is 'disturbed' by some 'symptom' or 'sign' (C-1 (h), lines 5-13). Also, the reader's knowledge of medicine is perceived as being limited: 'Regardless of what he himself may know of disease or disability, the patient should consult the doctor at the earliest sign . . .' (C-1 (h), lines 17-19).

Summary

The reader will note from the preceding section that the introductory discourses of the three textbooks are far more similar to one another with respect to editorial stance than are those of the popular books to one another. Firstly, the perceived function of all three textbooks is to perpetuate a tradition of medical education whose goal is the logical and systematic application of scientific medical knowledge to clinical practice. Secondly, the physician-editors in each case identify themselves with a tradition established by respected predecessors; and thirdly, the intended reader is always assumed to be either a member, or an anticipated member, of the medical profession.

In contrast, while the perceived function of popular books is the instruction of the reader, the editorial 'platform' varies considerably in each case (e.g. 'prevention', 'naturomatic healing', etc.). Moreover, attitudes towards physicians are inconsistent: he is variously seen as overworked and consequently negligent either in treating or communicating with his patients, as a vehicle of the miracles of medical science, as a prophet, or as an unassailable authority on the subject of disease. Finally, assumptions about the intended reader vary from book to book, not only with respect to his level of background knowledge, but also with respect to his economic status, his adherence or lack of adherence to traditional medical precepts, and his state of health.

This completes the semiotic analyses of all three segments of the eight selected books of medical instruction appearing in Part Two: (1) the Text (Part Two, II: 1), (2) the Table of Contents (Part Two, II: 2), and (3) the Paratext (Part Two: II: 3).

All tables, graphs, and supplements resulting from these analyses and appearing in Parts One and Two will subsequently be cited in Part Three in support of arguments demonstrating the ways in which textbooks of medicine differ from popular home medical books with respect to form and contents.

SUPPLEMENT C

C-1
Introductory Discourse

(a)   *T-1*
Preface

It is often asked why prefaces are written and whether they
are ever read. In his famous preface to *Cromwell,* Victor
Hugo pointed out that one seldom inspects the cellar of a
house after visiting its salons nor examines the roots of a
tree after eating its fruit. Admittedly, the readers of   5
this book will judge it by the substance of its contents
and its style, not by the pretexts offered by its editors.
It could be added that if the guest has returned several
times, then surely he knows that the cellar is well stocked.
Why then a preface to an eighth edition?   10
    This preface is intended to indicate the ways in which the
present edition maintains or diverges from, as the case may
be, the original objectives of this book. By doing this,
it will be possible to present the objectives of this textbook of medicine to readers unfamiliar with earlier editions.   15
    When the first group of editors met together almost thirty
years ago, they decided to write a textbook of medicine
which would conform to the *clinical method* which they had
found most useful both as students and as teachers. It
was thought that such a book should recapitulate the steps   20
in the process of thinking by which a physician reaches a
diagnosis, these being the recording of the patient's
symptoms and signs, the consideration of the various disorders that can give rise to them, and the effective
utilization of measures which will support and confirm   25
or alter the first impressions and lead ultimately to a
firm diagnosis.
    The logical first step consistent with this clinical
approach is the consideration of the cardinal manifestations of disease. Patients present themselves with   30
symptoms, not diagnoses. Consequently it is basic to
good clinical medicine to appreciate the different causes

of various manifestations of disease and to understand
how they may be produced. This requires an understanding
of physiology and of the ways in which deviations from   35
the normal lead to disorders of one kind or another. For
this reason material of fundamental biologic importance was
incorporated in the first edition of this book and has been
regarded as an essential component ever since.

The revolutionary changes in the curricula of many American   40
medical schools, particularly the abbreviation of the
standard courses in the science basic to clinical medicine
and the substitution of shorter 'core' courses, has im-
posed, we believe, additional responsibilities on the
modern teacher of clinical medicine and on the modern text-   45
book of medicine. The students who embark on their clinical
training now, although far more sophisticated in many ways
than their predecessors of even one generation ago, may not
possess as much understanding of the mechanisms of symptoms
and disease processes as is required to deal intelligently   50
with clinical problems. This book recognizes the challenge
to education posed by such curricula. Clinical biochemistry
and pathophysiology form an integral part of this book but,
insofar as possible, are considered within the clinical setting.

The interpretation of symptoms usually is most effectively   55
achieved by proceeding from the general to the particular.
Symptoms often can be grouped as syndromes. Syndromes are
the consequence of a variety of etiologic factors or
disease mechanisms and, if these can be recognized and
understood, measures to restore the normal physiologic   60
state can be designed and carried out in a logical, systematic fashion. Furthermore, the method of approaching a
diagnosis which is based on an analysis of the symptoms,
recognition of the syndrome, and consideration of the
various mechanisms which may have produced it, ensures   65
consideration of the many possible interpretations of the
clinical picture which the patient presents. By pursuing
such an approach, it is less likely that a disorder
which should be considered will be overlooked. The
problem-oriented record which is discussed in a special   70
chapter in this edition (Chap. 4) facilitates such a
logical approach to the consideration of the patient's complaints.

The plan of this book is consistent with this approach.

Following a discussion of the editors' general philosophy
regarding the approach to the patient (Part One), the   75
Cardinal Manifestations of Disease are considered (Part Two).
The mechanisms whereby various symptoms are produced are
discussed and an approach to the recognition of the diseases
of which they may be manifestations is outlined. Laboratory
findings are discussed in relation to the clinical manifes-   80
tations. Part Three summarizes important Biological Considerations in the Approach to Clinical Medicine and includes
sections on Genetics and Human Disease with a discussion of
cytogenetics, prenatal diagnosis, and genetic counselling;
Clinical Pharmacology with chapters on principles of drug   85
action and reactions to drugs; a section Metabolic Considerations which includes chapters on intermediary metabolism
of carbohydrate, fat, and protein, fluid and electrolytes,
acidosis and alkalosis; and a section on Immunologic
Considerations.   90
    The remainder of the book is concerned with specific dis-
orders and disease entities. In all these sections, the
syndromic approach is emphasized insofar as possible. The
reader will find at the beginning of most of the sections,
either in the introduction and/or in the first chapter, a   95
discussion of the approach to the patient whose clinical
manifestations suggest the type of disease considered in
that section.
    Treatment is discussed in relation to specific disorders or
categories of disease (e.g. Chapter 130, Chemotherapy of   100
Infection; Chapter 239, Pharmacologic Treatment of Cardiovascular Disorders) and is described in terms which are as
specific as practical.

. . . .

With the publication of the seventh edition of the Text-
book one of its original editors and Editor-in-Chief for   105
that edition, Dr. Maxwell M. Wintrobe, retired. Dr.
Wintrobe made major contributions to the Textbook over a
period of nearly thirty years, encompassing seven successive editions. It was Dr. Wintrobe and his associates in
Salt Lake City who sponsored the unique system of critical   110
review of each new chapter by *medical students* and *house*

staff as well as *faculty members,* thus giving the editors
very helpful insight as to the needs and ideas of the
'consumer'. Dr. Wintrobe's advice and counsel will be
missed, but his influence undoubtedly will continue to   115
be felt in succeeding editions of the Textbook.

GEORGE W. THORN
RAYMOND D. ADAMS
EUGENE BRAUNWALD
KURT J. ISSELBACHER
ROBERT G. PETERSDORF

(b)   *T-2*
Preface

This fourteenth edition of the Textbook of Medicine is
dedicated in warm and respectful affection to the memory
of Russell L. Cecil and Robert F. Loeb. Their influence
goes on in the essential character created and maintained
by them for the book and in the long-range effects they   5
have had as teachers and editors. Although their names no
longer appear on the title page, the book still carries
their imprint throughout.

    Each played a different yet essential part in the develop-
ment of this textbook. In the mid-1920s, Dr. Cecil had   10
the wisdom to perceive that a single-authored text in
medicine would no longer suffice and created the first
multiauthored textbook of medicine. Twenty years later
he had the further wisdom to perceive that the scientific
base of medicine had so enlarged that his own background   15
in science was no longer sufficiently contemporary. Hence
he invited Dr. Loeb to join him as coeditor. This
marriage of the private physician-professor and the full-
time academic professor was a very happy one; each com-
plemented the other perfectly. Both were dedicated to   20
the idea of getting the key concepts and useful practices
of the specialist and the scientist into a form that
could be employed by physicians and medical students.
Under the coeditorship of Dr. Loeb the textbook changed
subtly. It became less the repository of established   25

doctrine and more the expression of advanced, ongoing
ideas in medicine.

Dr. Cecil tended to worry more about the physician and
Dr. Loeb about the medical student; yet each was deeply
interested in both. Each had ample claims to distinction   30
quite aside from the book, and in the course of their long
careers, each benefited many people. It was their joint
editorial venture, however, that allowed them to exert a
healing influence on the many thousands of patients they
never got to see and a learning influence on the many   35
thousands of students who could not know personally their
extraordinary dedication to teaching. This lengthened
shadow is a very real part of their memorial and our legacy.

. . . .

By its tenth edition (1959) when this textbook had attained
world recognition and probably the widest use of any English   40
language textbook of medicine, Cecil and Loeb retired from
academic medicine and from their joint editorship. The
W. B. Saunders Company invited us to succeed them as co-
editors, and we gladly accepted with the goal of striving
to maintain the high standards set by our predecessors.   45

. . . .

There are 200 contributors to the present edition, of whom
72 are making contributions for the first time. In addition, a considerable number of contributors to previous
editions have elected to rewrite rather than simply re-
vise, so that fully half the present edition is assembled   50
from new manuscripts. As Editors, we have accepted responsibility for maintaining reasonable balance in the length
and style of contributions. In consultation with the expert editorial staff of the Saunders Company, we have again
given special attention to the headings of sections, chap-   55
ters, and paragraphs in order to make the book as easy to
use as possible. In the Table of Contents we have reverted
to a style employed in some of the earlier editions, which
we think makes for easier use than that in some more recent
editions. We have also introduced a system of cross-   60

reference by chapter, which is made easier by printing the
chapter number in the running head of each right-hand page.

A major goal in this edition has been to give as much
information as practical about therapy. Each contri-
butor has been specially requested to pay attention to   65
this point. Furthermore, we have introduced five new
chapters solely about treatment: Antimicrobial Therapy,
Cytotoxic and Immunosuppressive Agents, Medical Treatment
of Hormone-Dependent Cancers, Respiratory Failure and Its
Management, and Diet Therapy in Acute and Chronic Disease.   70
A new essay appears in Part I, dealing with Care of the
Patient with Terminal Illness. Various other areas in which
treatment is complex have been given additional space, e.g.,
management of renal insufficiency, management of shock and
heart failure, use of anticonvulsant drugs, treatment of
pain, and the problems of drug intoxication and addictions.   75

We view seriously our responsibility as custodians of what
has become a classic medical text during the past half
century; yet we realize full well that for the expert quality
of substance, it is the contributors who must be thanked.
We do this with gratitude.

PAUL B. BEESON
WALSH MC DERMOTT

(c)   *T-3*
Preface to the seventeenth edition

In 1892 the first edition of Sir William Osler's textbook
was published, in which he covered single-handedly the entire
field of medicine. His book was well received both as a
scientific work and as a contribution to literature. When
the time came for the seventh edition, he wrote the follow-   5
ing in a letter to Dr. Lewellys Barker: 'This new edition
will not be a very serious revision, as they will not break
up the plates, but in the next edition we can do as we like.
It would be very nice if you and Thayer came in with me as
joint authors. It would be possible, I think, to arrange   10
to have the work kept up as a Johns Hopkins Textbook of
Medicine'. This never came about. After Dr. Osler's death,

the textbook was edited by Dr. Thomas McCrae until the com-
pletion of the twelfth edition in 1935. After the death of
Dr. McCrae, Dr. Henry Christian continued as editor through   15
the sixteenth and last edition published in 1947.

This current revision was conceived as a Johns Hopkins Textbook of Medicine as proposed by Osler. There was hesitancy
to assume this task in view of the several excellent, comprehensive textbooks of medicine already available. However,   20
it was decided that there was a need for a different type
of textbook, one which would complement the existent encyclopedic texts. This text emphasizes clinical problems rather
than disease entities. It attempts to describe and define
the way in which the experienced physician approaches the   25
solution and management of such problems.

This is clearly not a revision of Dr. Osler's great book.
Nor is it the product of a single author. Rather, it is
the product of a single department in which the preservation
of a heritage of clinical excellence has been a major goal.   30
We hope this volume reflects the tradition of excellence
which this Department of Medicine received from Dr. Osler.

The Editors

Preface

In this Nineteenth Edition, the majority of the sections
have been completely revised, while a few have undergone   35
minor revisions and the factual information and the
bibliography brought up-to-date.

Since the last edition was published in 1972, several of the
authors have taken new positions in other medical schools.
In view of the fact that the basic theme of this textbook   40
has been the approach to medical practice as exemplified
by the staff of a single Department of Medicine, these
authors have been replaced by others who still remain or
have more recently come to Johns Hopkins.

. . . .

We also wish to thank all of our colleagues who have offered   45
constructive criticisms and whose advice in editing the
various sections has been of great help.

. . . .

The Editors

Foreword

In the practice of medicine the physician is confronted by
three basic questions: 50
   1. What is the matter with the patient?
   2. What can I do for him?
   3. What will be the outcome?
A fourth question, Why did it happen? will also arise in the
mind of the inquiring physician who feels that each patient   55
affords an opportunity and imposes a responsibility to contribute to a better understanding of causation and prevention.
   The usual textbook of medicine does not prepare the practitioner to deal systematically with these questions. Its
focus is upon the disease rather than the patient. It   60
presents its subject matter in a series of essays each
devoted to a description—as simple and straightforward as
possible—of the disease entity. Some general information
may be provided but rarely is sufficient emphasis placed
upon the confusing complexities which arise in the day-to-   65
day investigation and management of clinical problems.
The answer to the first of the questions enumerated above is
the key to the answers to the second and third. The first
question is the only one which requires an analytical approach,
and obviously the analysis must begin with a study of the   70
patient and must continue to be focused upon him until a
solution is reached.
   It is our purpose to produce a book which is built around
the patient rather than the disease—the patient and the
problems which he presents in diagnosis, management, and   75
prognosis. Consideration will be given to the methods
employed in acquiring factual data, the discriminating use
of ancillary diagnostic techniques, and the systematic
analysis of the accumulated information. This book also
presents the essential information necessary for an understanding of the basic mechanisms involved in the various   80
manifestations of disease, the important features of the
natural history of the major diseases, the principles

involved in the management of the patient, and the esti-
mation of the probable outcome. In order to devote more
space to the sequential steps which should be taken by the   85
physician seeking the answers to his three basic questions,
we have avoided as far as possible duplication of the type
of presentation so successfully employed in texts already
available. Since much of the material contained in current
texts is to be sacrificed, the physician may have to turn   90
elsewhere to fill the gaps in his knowledge of the subject
in hand. To meet this need for quick access to more detailed information on specific topics, particular attention has been devoted to the selection and cross-indexing
of the bibliography.   95

The Editors

(d)   *P-1*
Foreword

The Family Medical Guide has been in preparation over a
period of several years by a corps of medical men which
includes several of America's most distinguished specialists and authorities.
    We've designed the book to supplement the counsel of one's   5
own personal physician, who alone is competent to diagnose
and treat conditions in individual patients. Advances in
medicine make it more than ever necessary that intelligent
persons have some understanding of body structures and
processes of health and disease which doctors can rarely   10
take the time to explain fully to us.
    The Better Homes and Gardens Family Medical Guide is a
reference to which you may turn for authoritative information about health problems that arise from time to time
in your family and personal life, as well as about prac-   15
tical matters of appropriate home care, prevention of
disease, maintenance of health, and recognition of illness leading to prompt treatment by a physician who has
the great resources of modern medicine at his and your
disposal. The illustrations illuminate the wondrous   20
mechanisms of the body and they identify structures con-

cerned with particular conditions. We explain unfamiliar
technical terms; none have we avoided, as many 'doctor's
words' are now part of the common language.

Eminent physicians have demonstrated their belief that such   25
a book is desirable by taking time from their practices and
from their academic duties to contribute chapters on their
special fields of medicine. We invited each contributor to
discuss his topic as if he were speaking across his desk to
an intelligent and concerned patient and with all the time   30
in the world to give counsel and to dispel misconceptions.
Some of the topics are discussed by different specialists.
Cross-references throughout the book direct you to more
extended discussions. If this book helps to make you a
more understanding patient, then it's surely the indispen-   35
sable complement to an understanding doctor.

(e)   *P-2*
Foreword by a Doctor of Medicine

This book by a Doctor of Chiropractic deals with natural
self-help remedies that should be useful to persons of all
ages. It is now generally well known that good health depends upon good nutrition and good living habits. It is
also well known that there are a multitude of ailments that   5
are best cared for with simple, drugless remedies that are
within the reach of everyone. Natural remedies and natural
foods build good health, and they help to prevent diseases
and illnessses that shorten life.

The programs outlined in this book are based on natural laws   10
that form a common denominator for all healing methods, and
they represent a sincere effort to help people who want to
help themselves. No one can dispute the value of natural
foods, moist heat, and other natural techniques that should
be a part of every individual's effort to ease his aches and   15
pains and prolong his life.

You are personally responsible for your health and the care
of your body. You must read and study books such as this,
if you are to be knowledgeable enough to help yourself and
protect your health. You must be broad-minded in your   20
search for effective ways to care for your body. In the

final analysis, you alone must make the final judgement of
the effectiveness of remedies and measures that affect your
health.

This book by Samuel Homola describes many safe, simple   25
natural remedies and health-building measures that could
be recommended by any practitioner who is sincerely concerned about helping others. I therefore recommend this
book for all those who are searching for drugless remedies
that are designed to build health as well as relieve   30
suffering.

Jonathan Forman, B.A., M.D.,
F.A.C.A., F.I.C.A.N.

What this book can do for you

The average family spends several hundred dollars and upwards
each year on medical bills. Much of this may be spent for   35
simple, minor ailments that could be handled successfully
at home without professional care.

Unfortunately, few doctors have the time to tell their
patients how to help themselves. With illness so rampant
and doctors so overworked, only 'serious' disorders receive   40
adequate attention in the average doctor's office. The
truth is, however, that many 'minor' disorders can develop
into serious disease when they are neglected. And if they
aren't handled with natural healing methods that stimulate
the healing powers of the body, they may never be completely   45
cured.

There are millions of people who are suffering from minor and
chronic ailments that would respond immediately to properly
applied natural remedies. Few of these people are aware of
the fact that their suffering could be relieved at home.
What about you? Are you suffering from some nagging ailment   50
that makes your life miserable? Your body has a remarkable
capacity to heal itself when it is helped along by natural
healing methods.

In this book, I have outlined basic home-treatment methods
for a great variety of common and not-so-common ailments,   55
and I show you how to help your body heal itself naturally.
For less than the price of one office call, you can acquire

more health guidance from this book than a doctor could give
you in a hundred office calls—and the book is yours to keep
for the rest of your life. Regular use of this book will   60
cut down your health expenses, as well as tell you exactly
what to do to help yourself and relieve your suffering.
You can care for many of your ailments as effectively as the
most expensive specialist. You don't have to run to an
overworked doctor's office every time you have a muscle   65
spasm, a cold, or a headache.

Remember that *only nature heals.* Any treatment that may be
of value to you as a home remedy must aid nature without
harming your body. So don't confuse natural healing methods
with patent medicines that do nothing but choke off   70
symptoms. Some drugs actually *delay* healing by interfering
with the internal processes of the body. Natural remedies
improve body functions as a whole, thus improving your
health and prolonging your life.

With this book, you'll have a handy and easy-to-read guide   75
to reliable and effective natural remedies that can be used
by every member of your family. You'll learn how to handle
hundreds of ailments with tried and proven natural healing
methods that have produced prompt results for a great many
people. The home remedies in this book combine healing   80
science with 'folk medicine' and 'health secrets' in a
self-help program that I am confident will work as well
for you as it does for me and my patients.

There are several special features for your health benefit
in this book. As a practicing chiropractor, I'm able to   85
bring you many new methods of treatment that have not been
described, to the best of my knowledge, in books written
for laymen. A new spinal manipulation technique, for
example, that can be used safely at home by anyone, will do
wonders in relieving aches and pains that do not respond to   90
conventional treatment methods. Also, my work in training
and treating athletes enables me to bring you many new and
effective treatment methods that have been designed to
produce rapid and lasting results.

This is *not* one of those books that dwells only on nutrition,   95
body mechanics, or some other specialized method of healing.
This book tells you how to use *all* the natural remedies and
healing methods and how to apply them to *all* the ailments
that can be cared for at home.

However, if I had to give the methods in this book one all-   100
encompassing name, I would call them 'Naturomatic Healing',
because the whole system of natural healing which I describe
seems to work automatically to help your body heal itself,
and restore its natural health balance. Thus, each and every
technique mentioned in the book might be considered part of   105
the Naturomatic Healing Method.

Samuel Homola, D.C.

(f)   *P-3*[39]
The promise

There was a time when preventive medicine was—and could be—
only a hope. It was expressed in the custom of the ancient
Chinese who paid their doctors to keep them well; when they
became patients, they refused to pay. It was implicit in
the adage of ancient Greek medicine: 'Help your patients   5
to die young—as late as possible'.

. . . .

Recent decades have been great strides in curative medicine.
But the most significant developments now are not magic new
drugs and surgical procedures that cure but new insights into
how disease arises and, if present, prevented from pro-   10
gressing.

. . . .

Treatment never equals prevention. Treatment, the best that
can be devised, must be used when disease exists. But
treatment does not always work; even when it does, it may
eliminate the disease but not the damage already done. It   15
is prevention that must be counted upon to make the big
inroads against both death and disability.

. . . .

. . . a major share of the credit must go to the sanitary

engineer, the agriculturist, the public health officer, the
pediatrician, and the family physician practicing preven-   20
tive medicine. Nearly all the gains against the once-
great killers—which also included typhoid fever, smallpox,
plague—have been made as the result of improvements in
sanitation, in nutrition, in immunization procedures, and
in early diagnosis through mass disease screening campaigns—   25
all techniques of disease prevention.

Therapeutic measures, including the antibiotics and other
wonder drugs, have helped but not nearly as much as preventive measures. In fact, it has been observed that only
two major diseases in the United States today—appendicitis   30
and lobar pneumonia in the young—are being controlled rather
completely by treatment alone. Prevention has much more to
offer.

. . . .

The fact is, too, that as deaths in the early years of life
from infectious diseases have declined, the other disorders—   35
often called degenerative diseases and once regarded chiefly
as consequences of aging—have become important killers and
cripplers of people in the middle years and even earlier.
No longer, for example, are the heart attack and the stroke
solely the unwelcome companions of retirement; they are now   40
threats to life to people at the height of their careers.

As a result, there has been a change of attitude about these
diseases—from one of passive acceptance of their inevit-
ability to one of determined attack. Part of the attack, of
course, is a search for cures and palliative measures. But   45
the best hope for eliminating these disorders lies in preventing their occurrence. And the most promising aspect of
the attack is the emergence of a new kind of preventive
medicine, broader-based but also individualized.

The Three Stages of Prevention   50
. . . .

The ideal is to prevent disease, if possible, from happening.
But the new preventive medicine, on a realistic basis, also
includes secondary prevention: the prevention, if a disease

is already present, of progression. It also includes ter- 55
tiary prevention: the holding in check of even far-advanced
disease so that radical measures, such as organ substitution
when applicable, may be used.

Implicit, too, in the new preventive medicine is a positive
aspect: an improvement in the quality of living as well as
length of life, a building of physical, mental, and emo- 60
tional health.

We Americans, a warmhearted people, like to rally round to
'help the handicapped'—and we think of the handicapped as
the blind, crippled, mentally deficient. Yet many of us,
although free of such obvious deficits, belong among the 65
handicapped.
If not outrightly sick, we are never fully healthy. We live
in 'second gear'. One dramatic large-scale demonstration of
this came in World War II when many relatively young men, in
their early thirties and even twenties, had to be rejected
by the Armed Forces as unfit. We have current reminders of 70
our state of non-first-class health in the daily barrages
of 'remedy' advertising on television—all the concoctions
offering relief for tired feelings, stomach upsets, heartburn, acid indigestion, insomnia, tension, a multitude of
aches and pains. 75

Is vigorous health impossible? It should be the rule rather
than the exception—and at older ages as well as earlier life.

Man may or may not have the capacity for living to 150 or
200 years of age; there is considerable debate about this in
medical circles. And there is not yet in sight any medical 80
ability to bring a halt to aging. But with knowledge now
available, the aging process can be slowed. Indeed, a good
deal of what is passed off as deterioration due to aging
is not that at all; it is deterioration due to insult or
neglect. And preventive medicine has much to offer in 85
showing how the insult and neglect can be eliminated.

The goals are ambitious, and certainly much more research
is needed before they are fully—and universally—attain-
able and their necessity generally accepted. But already
enough research has been done, enough tools have been de- 90
veloped, and the tactics have become sufficiently clear to
make the new preventive medicine a practical matter for
you and your family.

To help make it so is, of course, our aim in writing this
book. We have tried to provide in it a detailed guide to   95
the concepts and practices of preventive medicine—how
the physician uses them and how the individual can apply them.

THE TACTICS

'To cure sometimes, to relieve often, to comfort always'—
so the physician's role was described in the fifteenth   100
century. So it remained until this century. Comfort he
did because there was little else he could do.
Twentieth-century medicine has undergone fundamental changes,
with more progress made in a few decades than in thousands   105
of years before. And while some of this progress has been
dramatically obvious—heart surgery, brain surgery, antibiotics, hormonal treatments—even more basic advances were
being made at the same time.
    Medicine began to penetrate the mysteries of psychic disease   110
and to gain understanding of the interrelationships of mind
and body. It explored the influence and mechanisms of heredity in disease. It established the mechanisms of body
chemistry and of inborn chemical error. It allied itself
with many other sciences—drawing, for example, from physics   115
and biochemistry new electronic equipment and test tube
procedures for detecting and monitoring disease.
    The crystal ball may seem less glamorous than the wonder
drug and the miracle in the operating room. But medicine
has been developing a kind of scientific crystal ball that   120
promises to make far greater inroads on disease, that can
be rubbed to see the portents for the individual patient
and used to help guide him around the health hazards he
faces.

Calculating risks   125

First, it became evident not only that people vary in
susceptibility to disease but that increased risk depends
upon many factors and that it is possible to calculate risks.
    Breast cancer, for example, occurs in 5 percent of white
women over age 40 in the United States—and so, on the   130
average, there is a 1 in 20 risk. But a woman with a
positive family history of breast cancer—one whose mother

or sister or aunt developed the disease—has triple the
risk of other women. (Let us say, at once, that if this
increased hazard because of hereditary influences stood by   135
itself, it would be only a morbid statistic. But it stands
with increasingly sensitive methods of detecting cancer at
earlier and earlier—and therefore more curable—stages, and
underscores the wisdom of special emphasis on breast cancer
detection for such a woman.)   140
    Other factors, racial and social, help to identify special
pronenesses. The Japanese have a high risk of stomach cancer
but relatively low risk of breast cancer; the Chinese and
Malaysians have a high risk of nose and throat cancer. In
unskilled American workers and their wives, the incidence   145
of cancer of the stomach and uterine cervix is three to four
times higher than among people in the professional fields.
On the other hand, cancer of the breast and leukemia are
substantially more common in the higher economic classes.
    There are occupational factors to be considered. For example,   150
urinary bladder cancer has an increased incidence among aniline dye workers, and in that industry programs have been
started for annual tests of urine.

. . . .

Disease scenarios

Another important development has been the discovery that
death is really a slow intruder, that diseases do not   155
suddenly spring up full-blown but often have long scenarios.
    In the Korean War, autopsies of young American soldiers re-
vealed that in 54 percent of these youths, many of whom had
only very recently attained manhood, coronary heart disease
was already starting. No longer could the disease be con-   160
sidered degenerative, a part of aging. If the seeds of the
disease germinate in the early years and the ultimate heart
attack is the end result of a long process in time, then
here is a problem that can be combatted, for there is time
to combat it. And since there is evidence of what factors   165
are involved, there are means to fight, to retard, and
perhaps even to prevent it from getting started.

. . . .

How does a preventively minded physician function?

You can expect that in working with you he will get to know
you thoroughly—past medical history, family medical his-   170
tory, job, working habits, living habits—so he can weigh
any possibility that you—as a member of a specific group
based on heredity, environment, age, sex, color, personal
habits—may face certain specific health hazards.

In his regular periodic examinations, he will follow your   175
health progress in general and will be alert for the
slightest early indication of anything wrong in any area of
special risk for you. He may, in fact, from time to time
use special tests to make certain all is going well in a   180
special risk area.

During your visits, he will be concerned, of course, with
any physical complaints and also with any mental or emotional problems (job, marital, and others), since these can
affect health.   185

He will be interested in any changes in your habits and their
possible effects, for good or ill, on your health. From
time to time, he may have suggestions for an alteration,
perhaps minor, of diet, exercise pattern, sleep, relaxation, etc.   190

As he regularly checks you, alert for earliest indications,
even preindications, of possible trouble, he will be prepared to intervene without delay. Rather than wait, say,
for obvious symptoms of diabetes to develop—especially
if you belong to the group with greater than average   195
probability of developing the disease—he will intervene
to try to correct, if they appear, the very first changes
that could possibly lead to diabetes.

As medicine has been practiced generally to now, it has been
the patient who, in effect, has turned up after making a   205
self-diagnosis. It has been the patient who has decided,
'I think I am or may be sick or becoming sick', and then
has sought help.

Now it will be the preventively minded physician who increasingly will be able to tell the patient; 'You are about to   210
become sick and we are going to take a few measures in advance so you won't actually develop the sickness'.

(g) *P-4*
Introduction

The world of science as it relates to health has moved rapidly
since the publication of the first edition of *The Encyclopedia
of Common Diseases.* In the '60s alone, hearts were trans-
planted, the Pill passed into common usage, scores of environmental causes of cancer were identified, nutritional therapy   5
for emotional disturbances earned new respect and hundreds
of other changes in our attitudes toward disease became commonplace. In terms of health, the years since World War II
have brought the civilized world into a whole new era.

    The rapidity with which this new era in medicine has developed   10
explains why the material in this edition is more than 75 percent new. Some subjects, such as crib death and venereal
disease, did not appear in the original at all. Others, such
as Emotional and Nervous Disorders and Back Ailments, have
been greatly expanded. Some sections, particularly those on   15
the heart and cancer, are books in themselves.

    Each disease section has been carefully researched for the
latest information and all medical and scientific conclusions
are based on reports from the most respected of the world's
medical and scientific journals.   20

    Obviously, in the face of serious illness no book, however
thorough it might be, can take the place of a consultation
with a physician. However, the informed patient understands,
more readily, the symptoms of his illness and the aims of
the treatment. Furthermore, he is prepared to ask the doc-   25
tor the right questions and volunteer important information
that can help in his treatment.

    Every person is responsible for his own health. He must
learn how his body works and what can threaten its functioning. The person who identifies these threats and tries to   30
avoid them is taking the most important steps there are in
battling disease. This book outlines these steps in a useful, understandable manner.

    The underlying philosophy of *The New Encyclopedia of Common
Diseases* is 'natural is best'. This means that when there   35
is solid scientific evidence that drugless, nonsurgical
treatments have proven effective, they are emphasized.

    Of course, some ailments allow no time for experimentation

with home remedies. For example, pneumonia, heart attack
or appendicitis demand immediate medical attention. The   40
miraculous advances medical science has made show to their
best advantage at such times. But as a rule, health comes
from the way people live, not from doctors and hospitals.
This book is a blueprint for better, more healthful living.

(h)   *P-5*
Preface

Many new discoveries have been developed in medical science
with relationship to some of the diseases that are discussed
in this book. Some subjects insufficiently discussed in
previous issues have been given more consideration.
    When people come to a doctor, they usually come because   5
they have had pain or some other symptom which has continued to disturb them, or which has not been explained.
The pain may be headache, stomach ache, or pain elsewhere
in the body like the pains of rheumatoid arthritis. People
consult the doctor because of sudden or extreme loss of   10
weight, or unexplained fever, or similar conditions. For
any unexplainable condition, the person should consult the
doctor at the earliest sign. The modern doctor will attempt
to solve the condition through a complete examination which
will include not only attention to the special pain or symp-   15
tom or disturbance, but also tests to detect any condition
in the body that needs attention. Regardless of what he
himself may know of disease or disability, the patient should
consult the doctor at the earliest sign, and he should be
prepared to have his condition approached from the point of   20
view of his whole body. This may necessitate a study which
requires the use of the X-ray, or a variety of laboratory
examinations, of a record of all of his previous diseases,
and a most intimate search into the condition for which he
consults a physician.   25
    This book, it is hoped, will give the reader a better under-
standing of his own medical troubles and thereby make him
a better patient for his doctor.

Morris Fishbein, M.D.

Chicago

C-2
Dedications

T-1
To all those who have taught us, and especially to our younger colleagues who continue to teach and inspire us

T-2

Dedicated to the memory of
Russell L. Cecil, 1881-1965
and
Robert F. Loeb, 1895-1973
Great teachers of medicine
who in their editorial partnership were able
to better the lives of thousands more patients
and students than they ever got to see

T-3
This volume is dedicated to the physicians of the Medical Service of the past for their precept and guidance, to our colleagues of today for their support and encouragement, and to the students, our colleagues of tomorrow, for their stimulation and criticism

P-1   0

P-2
Dedicated to my father, the late Dr. Joseph Homola

P-3

To
Judith W. Miller
and
Barbara Galton
our wives
who gave us the time
and encouragement
to complete this book

P-4   0

P-5

Dedicated to
MY GRANDCHILDREN
Morris Fishbein, Merriel Anna, Peter Emil, and Rosemary Friedell
and to
Georgia Emily, Lawrence Victor, Michael Morris,
and the twins—Barbara Ann and Wendy Jo Marks
and to
Amy Louise, Morris Daniel, and Ann Marie Fishbein

C-3
Warnings Concerning Drug Administration and Therapy

T-1

Medicine is an ever-changing science. As new research and clinical experience broaden our knowledge, changes in treatment and drug therapy are required. The editors and the publisher of this work have made every effort to ensure that the drug dosage schedules herein are accurate and in accord with the standards accepted at the time of publication. Readers are advised, however, to check the product information sheet included in the package of each drug they plan to administer to be certain that changes have not been made in the recommended dose or in the contraindications for administration. This recommendation is of particular importance in regard to new or infrequently used drugs.

T-2   0

T-3

NOTICE. Our knowledge in the clinical sciences is constantly changing. As new information becomes available, changes in treatment and in the use of drugs becomes necessary. The contributors and the publisher of this volume have, as far as it is possible to do so, taken care to make certain that the doses of drugs and schedules of treatment are correct and compatible with the standards generally accepted at the time of publication. The physician or student is advised to consult carefully the instruction and information material included in the package insert of each drug or therapeutic agent that he plans to administer in order to make certain that the recommended dosage is correct and that there have been no changes in the recommended dose of the drug or in the indications or contraindications in its utilization. This advice is especially important when using new or infrequently used drugs.

P-1   0

P-2   0

P-3   0

P-4   0

P-5   0

C-4
Recent Translations

T-1

Foreign Editions: French (Seventh Edition)
Italian (Seventh Edition)
Polish (Fifth Edition)
Portuguese (Seventh Edition)
Spanish (Sixth Edition)
Turkish (Sixth Edition)·
Japanese (Seventh Edition)
Greek (Sixth Edition)

T-2

Portuguese (Thirteenth Edition)
Serbo-Croat (Eleventh Edition)
Spanish (Thirteenth Edition)

T-3
P-1
P-2
P-3   } none cited
P-4
P-5

NOTES

1. The reader is reminded that the term 'Text' is always to be understood in its technical sense (see Part Two, Section I: 4).
2. For definition, see Part Two, Section I: 4. For examples, see Supplement A-2.
3. The method of analysis of semantic fields or domains was developed by the German, J. Trier.

   'This method makes it possible to demonstrate that the articulation of a given notional region may vary according to the language or to the successive states of a single language'. (Oswald Ducrot and Todorov Tzvetan, *Encyclopedic Dictionary of the Sciences of Lanugage* (Baltimore: Johns Hopkins University Press, 1979), p. 135.

   'In recent years, there has been a good deal of work devoted to the investigation of lexical systems in the vocabularies of different languages, with particular reference to such fields (or domains) as kinship, color, flora and fauna, weights and measures, military ranks . . . and *various kinds of knowledge, skill, and understanding'.* (Lyons, *Introduction to Theoretical Linguistics,* Cambridge: Cambridge University Press, 1968), p. 429 (my emphasis). One such field or domain of 'knowledge, skill, and understanding' is the domain of Medicine.
4. 'Diabetes and its complications are now thought to be the third leading cause of death in the U.S., trailing only cardiovascular disease and cancer. According to a report issued by the National Commission on Diabetes in 1976, as many as 10 million Americans, or close to 5 percent of the population, may have diabetes, and the incidence is increasing yearly'. (Abner Louis Notkins, 'The causes of diabetes', *Scientific American* 241 [November 1979]: 62).
5. 'The earliest description of its symptoms is found in the Ebers papyrus of Egypt, dating back to 1500 B.C.' (Notkins 1979: 62)
6. Each Table has been provided with, and is followed by, a companion Graph bearing the same number as the Table, in which the data are presented in a more 'visually communicative' manner. I am grateful to Professor George Styan, of the Department of Mathematics of McGill University, for having introduced me to the 'stem-and-leaf' style of presenting data which has been used in all of the Graphs throughout this study. See also John W. Tukey, *Exploring Data Analysis* (Reading, Mass.: Addison-Wesley, 1977), p. 7.
7. Richard D. Mallery, *Grammar, Rhetoric, and Composition* (New York: Doubleday, 1967), p. 71.
8. Mallery 1967: 74.
9. Intersentential markers of coherence appear either at, or near, the beginning of sentences, and serve specifically to link sentences with one another. They include the following examples: thus, therefore, however, moreover, on the one hand (other hand), firstly, in addition, also, furthermore, nevertheless, still, likewise, conversely, despite this, hence, by contrast, consequently, accordingly, in summary, finally, etc.
10. Personal pronouns include the following: I, you, he, she, we, they, me, him, her, them, us, myself, yourself, himself, herself, themselves, mine, yours, his, hers, ours, theirs, my, your, her, our, their.
11. These terms have been verified as such by consulting Albert L.. Lehninger, *Biochemistry,* 2nd ed. (New York: Worth Publishers, 1977).
12. Type A terms contain the semantic component, 'one who is sick'. Thus 'patient(s)'

and 'diabetic(s)' are Type A terms. All other terms for human subjects are called Type B terms.

13. Two subclasses of Type B terms have been identified: Type B_1 terms which refer to all roles defined by age, sex, family membership, and occupation (i.e. biosocially defined roles), and Type B_2 terms, which include the terms 'person(s)' and 'people'.

14. On the subject of Schemata, the following passage provides an interesting historical perspective: 'Osler introduced a system for the description of disease which has been followed by many subsequent textbooks of medicine. It began with a definition, followed by a historical note, and discussions, in order, of etiology, transmission (for infectious diseases), morbid anatomy symptoms, diagnosis, prognosis, prophylaxis, and treatment' (Abner McGehee Harvey and Victor McKusick, *Osler's Textbook Revisited,* (New York: Appleton, 1967), p. 7.

    Also see Appendix E (a) for Osler's schema of diabetes mellitus from a 1909 edition of T-3.

15. The term 'mapping' has been borrowed from the field of mathematics, and will be used here (in a less strict sense) to indicate the procedure of matching a set of words from one heading with a set of words in another heading because of an identified semantic correlation between them.

    The criterion for mapping a set of bold-type headings from any of the eight Schemata into the set of chapter headings from *Joslin's* is as follows: that the semantic components of the former 'overlap', in a significant manner, with the semantic components of the latter, as corroborated by reference to (a) *Stedman's Medical Dictionary,* 23rd edition, and (b) *The Shorter Oxford English Dictionary on Historical Principles,* 3rd edition.

    To 'overlap in a significant manner' means that the relationship between at least one important lexical item in a bold-type heading, and at least one important lexical item in a chapter heading must be either one of identity (same orthographic form and same meaning), of synonymy (different orthographic form but same meaning), a class relation, or a part-to-whole relation. In certain cases, the justification for mapping bold-type headings into chapter headings may become apparent only if the reader refers as well to Appendix F (a), a supplement to the 'standard', in which appear *all* bold-type headings interspersed throughout the 32 chapters of *Joslin's.*

    Insofar as Appendix F (a) represents a *textbook* devoted exclusively to diabetes mellitus, it may interest the reader to compare it with Appendix F (b), which represents a *popular book* devoted exclusively to the same topic. In the writer's opinion, this comparison highlights very well some of the radical differences between textbook and popular approaches to the same subject.

16. Such sentences constitute 31% of all sentences in textbook descriptions, and 37% of all sentences in popular descriptions.

17. In addition to sentences where the pragmatic instruction is explicit, there are, of course, many other sentences (not included in this investigation) where the instruction is only implied.

18. As a group, these sentences are distinguished by the fact that they contain a variety of popular metaphors, slogans, cliches, quoted testimonials, malapropisms, paradoxes, hyperbolic statements, alliterative constructions, elliptical forms, and other markers of an informal style. Such markers have been underlined in the above examples. Since these kinds of sentences are exclusive to the popular Disease Descriptions, they have not been quantified.

Textbook descriptions were found to contain a number of *apparent* metaphors applied to the description of certain anatomical structures and physiological functions. However, since these were subsequently discovered to have been already included in *Stedman's Medical Dictionary* (23rd edition), they must, on that account, be considered as *dead* metaphors.

19. These kinds of sentences possibly have the effect of dispelling anxiety in the reader insofar as they: (1) de-emphasize the negative consequences of having the disease, (2) emphasize that there is much that the reader himself, through such 'natural' means as diet, dietary supplements, and the proper mental attitude, can do to preserve his health, and (3) inspire trust in the medical profession or in some of its pharmacological and technological advances. Since these kinds of sentences are found exclusively in popular Disease Descriptions, they have not been quantified.

20. Such terms for subdomains of medicine as 'immunology', 'cardiology', 'endocrinology', 'gastroenterology', etc. may be said to be related paradigmatically, i.e. 'all the members of the sets of semantically-related terms can occur in the same context' (Lyons 1968: 428). Headings in the Tables of Contents of textbooks more readily lend themselves to paradigmatic substitutions than do the headings in Tables of Contents of popular books.

21. It will become evident through the subsequent comparison between the Tables of Contents of textbooks and popular books, that the classificatory principle which informs the former group of books is, in contrast to the latter, almost exclusively 'nosological', i.e. concerned with the classification of diseases: 'A classification of diseases may be defined as a system of categories to which morbid entities are assigned according to some established criteria. There are many possible choices for these criteria. The anatomist, for example, may desire a classification based on the part of the body affected whereas the pathologist is primarily interested in the nature of the disease process, the public health practitioner in aetiology and the clinician in the particular manifestation requiring his care. In other words, there are many axes of classification and the particular axis will be determined by the interest of the investigator' (WHO *Manual,* p. vii).

22. Exceptions are the Tables of Contents of T-1, T-3, and P-3, from which (for reasons that will later be explained) certain subheadings have been selected as well.

23. An assumption is made that the linguistic properties of these main lexical items are very likely to be representative of the linguistic properties of main lexical items distributed throughout the Text.

24. The reader will recall that an 'external standard' was also recruited in the cross-comparison of Schemata.

25. WHO *Manual,* P. 1.

26. See note 15 for explanation of the term 'mapping procedure'.

27. That there are 16 rather than 17 sets of lexical items is attributable to the fact that the mapping procedure excluded 'Category XVI, Symptoms, Signs and Ill-defined Conditions'. See note b in Supplement B-1 (a), p. 144.

28. In the field of 'scientometrics', the numbers of certain kinds of lexical items in an Index of a scientific book are taken as indications of the conceptual focus of that book, and are compared historically with the Indexes of earlier scientific books as a means of 'measuring' conceptual trends in science. See Francis Narin, *Evaluative Bibliometrics: The Use of Publication and Citation Analysis in the Evaluation of Scientific Activity* (Cherry Hill, N.J.: Computer Horizons, 1976). Such a technique, in the opinion of the writer, could be applied as well to the measurement of conceptual trends in medical science.

29. All samples of introductory discourse (or relevant portions thereof) are to be found in Supplement C-1, pp. 199-219.
30. See Supplement C-1 (a), pp. 199-202.
31. See Supplement C-1 (b), pp. 202-204.
32. See Supplement C-1 (c), pp. 204-207.
33. See Supplement C-1 (d), pp. 207-208.
34. See Supplement C-1 (e), pp. 208-211.
35. 'No one can dispute the value of natural foods, moist heat, and other natural techniques . . .' (p. 208, lines 13-14).
36. See Supplement C-1 (f), pp. 211-214.

PART THREE

Conclusions

Differences in Form

Differences between textbooks and popular books with respect to form have been determined from four perspectives:

1. the distribution of nondiscursive elements;
2. the distribution of certain grammatical and other semiotic elements;
3. the distribution of Paratextual components;
4. differences in style.

1. NONDISCURSIVE ELEMENTS[1]

A cross-comparison of certain nondiscursive elements in all books indicates significant differences in their relative distribution in textbooks and popular books. These differences are displayed in Table 59 and its Graph which follow.

From Table 59 and its companion Graph, we may conclude the following:

(a) The average number of pages in the Texts of textbooks is almost three times greater than the average number of pages in the Texts of popular books (1,929 as compared to 655).

(b) Textbooks, on the average, have more citations per page (1.6 as compared to 0.006), more contributors per page (0.08 as compared to 0.01), and more illustrations per page (0.3 as compared to 0.1).

(c) 100% of textbook contributors are M.D.s as compared to 75% of popular contributors.

2. DIFFERENCES IN THE DISTRIBUTION OF CERTAIN GRAMMATICAL AND OTHER SEMIOTIC ELEMENTS[2]

Analyses of Disease Descriptions[3] (from the Texts) and of Selected Headings[4] (from the Tables of Contents) show that, in comparison to popular books, textbooks have relatively more of the following:

Table 59.   *Distribution of nondiscursive elements: Textbooks vs popular books*

	T-1	T-2	T-3	Total	Avge	P-1	P-2	P-3	P-4	P-5	Total	Avge
No. of pages in each text	2089	1893	1805	5787	1929	856	235	656	1274	256	3277	655
No. of citations in each text	2955	3756	2426	9137	3046	29	0	a	a	0	29	6
No. of contributors for each text	195	199	85	479	160	31	1	2	6	1	41	8
No. of contributors with M.D.s	195	199	85	479 (100%)		29	0	1	0	1	31 (76%)	6
No. of illustrations in each text	624	521	777	1922	641	516	8	10	0	19	553	111
Citation/page ratio	1.4	2	1.3	—	1.6	0.03	0	0	0	0	—	0.006
Contributor/page ratio	0.09	0.11	0.05	—	0.08	0.04	0.004	0.003	0.005	0.004	—	0.01
Illustration/page ratio	0.3	0.3	0.4	—	0.3	0.6	0.03	0.02	0	0.07	—	0.1

[a] In P-3 and P-4, citations are interspersed throughout the Text, and have not been counted.

Graph 59.
(a) *Citation/page ratio: individual values*   (b) *Contributor/page ratio: individual values*   (c) *Illustration/page ratio: individual values*

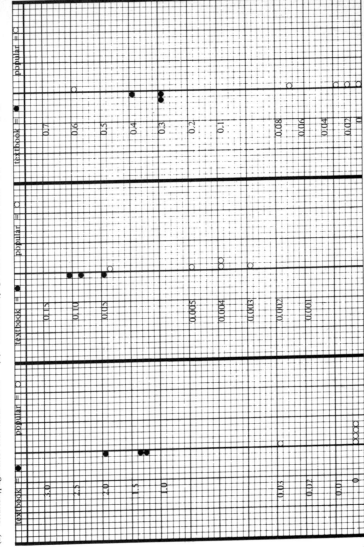

(a)   Lengthy sentences (DD: 24.3 words per sentence as compared to 20.4 words per sentence—see Table 2*).[5]

(b)   Simple sentences (DD: 53% as compared to 49%—see Table 3*).[6]

(c)   Assertive sentences (DD: 99.5% as compared to 93.8%—see Table 5*).

(d)   Prepositional phrases (SH: 19% as compared to 6%—see Table 45*).

(e)   Intersentential markers of coherence (DD: 0.5% as compared to 0.3%—see Table 6*).

(f)   Quantifications expressed in Arabic numerals (DD: 1.3% as compared to 0.4%—see Table 15*).

(g)   Bracketed constructions containing synonyms, explanations, etc. (DD: 0.5% as compared to 0.1%—see Table 16*).

(h)   Enumerated sets of words, phrases, etc. (DD: 0.05% as compared to 0.02%—see Table 17*).

(i)   Citations of works by other authors (DD: 0.2% as compared to 0.1%—see Table 18*).

In comparison to textbooks, popular books have relatively more of the following:

(a)   Short sentences (DD: 20.4 words per sentence as compared to 24.3 words per sentence—see Table 2*).

(b)   Nonsimple sentences (DD: 51% as compared to 47%—see Table 3*).

(c)   Nonassertive sentences (DD: 6.2% as compared to 0.5%—see Table 5*).

(d)   Adverbial clauses containing an infinitive (SH: 2% as compared to 0%—see Table 46*).

(e)   Monosyllabic words (SH: 28% as compared to 5%—see Table 41*).

(f)   Personal pronouns (DD: 1.6% as compared to 0.2%—see Table 7*, p. 86; and SH: 3% as compared to 0%—see Table 42*).

(g)   Compound nouns (SH: 10% as compared to 5%—see Table 44*).

(h)   Gerunds (SH: 4% as compared to 0%—see Table 43*).

3.   DIFFERENCES IN PARATEXTUAL COMPONENTS

Paratextual components found in all eight books of medical instruction have been listed and displayed in Table 58.

Three classes of these components may be demonstrated: Class T (exclusive to textbooks), Class P (exclusive to popular books), and Class T ∩ P (common to both).

Class T
1. List of Editors of Previous Editions
2. Warning Concerning Drug Administration and Therapy
3. Information Concerning Number of Recent Translations

Class P
1. Separate Acknowledgements (i.e. not part of the introductory discourse)
2. Glossary of Medical Terms
3. List of Other Books by Author or Editor
4. Photograph of Author or Editor (plus biographical data)

Class T ∩ P
1. Introductory Discourse (Preface, Foreword, or Introduction)
2. Appendix
3. Dedication
4. Index
5. List of Contributors and their Credentials

In Supplement C-2 the reader will note that in the case of popular books, dedications are addressed to members of the author's family, unlike in textbooks, where dedications are addressed to coprofessionals. Moreover, unlike textbooks, popular books include in their Paratextual components (a) a list of other books by the author or editor, and (b) a photograph (plus biographical data) of the author or editor (see Class P above). These facts suggest that the popular writer views his work more as the expression of an individual than as the contribution of a representative spokesman of a professional group.

4.   DIFFERENCES IN STYLE[7]

a.   *Textbook style*

Textbook style may be typified as (i) formal and (ii) authoritative (as distinct from popular style, which may be typified as informal and authoritarian).

(i)   Compared to popular style, textbook style may be called formal insofar as it is relatively more [a] systematic, [b] coherent, [c] precise, [d] uniform and [e] impersonal.[8]
   [a]   Textbook discourse is more systematic than popular discourse in that it provides relatively more bracketed constructions containing

explanations, synonyms, and examples (DD: 0.4% as compared to 0.1%—see Table 16), and relatively more enumerated sets of words, phrases, and sentences (DD: 0.05% as compared to 0.02%—see Table 17).

[b]   Textbook discourse is more coherent than popular discourse in that it contains relatively more intersentential markers of coherence (DD: 0.5% as compared to 0.3%—see Table 6).

[c]   Textbook discourse is more precise than popular discourse in that it contains relatively more numerical quantifications[9] (DD: 1.3% as compared to 0.4%—see Table 15).

[d]   Textbook discourse is more uniform than popular discourse, the characteristic sentence type being lengthy (DD: 24.3 words per sentence as compared to 20.4 words per sentence—see Table 2), assertive (DD: 99.5% as compared to 93.8%—see Table 5), and composed of numerous polysyllabic words (SH: 95% as compared to 72%—see Table 41). See also Supplement A-1.

[e]   Textbook style is more impersonal than popular style in that textbooks contain relatively fewer personal pronouns (DD: 0.2% as compared to 1.6%—see Table 7, and SH: 0% as compared to 3%—see Table 42).

(ii)   Compared to the style of popular books, textbooks may be called authoritative, hence more accountable. This characteristic of accountability is a product of the following factors:

[a]   Published research by other writers working in the same field are cited more frequently in textbooks than in popular books (DD: 0.2% as compared to 0.1%—see Table 18). Hence the discourse is located within a critical tradition.[10]

[b]   Standardized biomedical terminology is more frequently employed in textbooks than in popular books (DD: 4.5% as compared to 2.6%—see Table 8). Further evidence may be seen as well in comparing the terminology used in Schemata of textbooks vs popular books (See Tables 21 to 28). See also Appendix F for external confirmation of this general trend. Since the consistent use of such terminology diminishes the possibility of ambiguous interpretation by the reader, those statements expressed in such terminology will tend to be more accountable than will be statements expressed in terminology which is less specific with respect to meaning.

[c]   In textbooks, the territory of 'expertise' claimed by each author or editor is considerably more modest than is the case in popular books. Firstly, the number of authors per Disease Description is relatively higher in textbooks than in popular books (DD: 1.7% as compared to

1%—see Table 19). Secondly, the ratio of the average number of authors per Disease Description to the average number of contributors per book is considerably lower in textbooks than in popular books (1% as compared to 54%—see Table 19). Thirdly, it is of interest to note that while the chief editors of all three textbooks have achieved considerable academic distinction (see Appendix C), they have, on the average, edited or authored (or coedited or coauthored) far fewer books than is the case of the popular writers (see Appendix D, especially Table 60), of whom none of the latter (with the exception of the author of P-5) has achieved comparable academic distinction.

[d]   Editors of textbooks are held accountable by their coprofessionals, some of whom are assigned the task of reviewing and criticizing the works which they have edited (see Appendix B). Such reviews appear in journals devoted to the medical sciences (see Table 1), and are thereby accessible to wide professional readership. Insofar as such journals provide a common 'forum' within which a textbook may be corrected by informed coprofessionals (i.e. either the reviewer himself or else the journal readers), they help guarantee a high level of scholarly accountability with respect to future editions of that textbook.[11]

In contrast, reviews of popular books appear in a number of non-(medical) professional reviewing publications (see Table 1), and are written by laymen. Since it is unlikely that the majority of readers of such reviews possesses sufficiently high levels of medical knowledge to engage in informed criticism (i.e. criticism directed toward commonly-understood and precisely-defined issues), it is further unlikely that readership 'feedback' would have an effect upon the level of scholarity of subsequent editions of the reviewed book. Thus, because locations of popular reviews (such as newspapers and popular periodicals) do not create as rigorous a critical forum as do the journal locations of textbooks, the potential for popular books to be as accountable as textbooks is considerably diminished.

[e]   Finally, since textbook discourse exists within the context of a long publishing history of works which have all borne the same title, it is suggested that textbook writers are under certain constraints with respect to historical accountability. This would not be the case with the popular writers, in that all five popular books have much shorter 'genealogies' (see Graph 1; see also Appendix A).

b.   *Popular style*

Popular style may be described as (i) informal and (ii) authoritarian (as distinct from textbook style, which has been characterized as formal and authoritative).

(i)   Compared to textbook style, popular style may be called informal for the following reasons:

[a]   Popular books more frequently display certain informal grammatical constructions, such as contractions (e.g. 'it's, 'there's', and 'here's') as well as sentences beginning with the conjunctions 'but' and 'and' (see Supplement A-3).

[b]   The general tone in popular books, in contrast to textbooks, is personal, attributable largely to a relatively higher distribution of personal pronouns (DD: 1.6% as compared to 0.2%—see Table 7 and SH: 3% as compared to 0%—see Table 42).

[c]   The sentences found in popular discourse are less uniform in their construction than sentences found in textbook discourse. Whereas the majority of sentences both in textbook and popular discourse are of the assertive type, popular discourse contains a higher percentage of non-assertive sentences (DD: 6.2% as compared to 0.5%—see Table 5).

[d]   Popular books contain relatively more monosyllabic words than do textbooks (SH: 28% as compared to 5%—see Table 41), a feature which, in conjunction with the use of shorter sentences (see Table 2), contributes to the informal tone.

[e]   Finally, popular discourse contains many examples of colloquialisms of various types, as may be seen in Supplement A-3.

(ii)   Popular style may be called authoritarian, hence, low in accountability, for the following reasons:

[a]   Despite the fact that three of the five popular books (P-1, P-3, and P-5) have been written by physicians (see Table 59) and one of the five (P-2) by a chiropractor, the only popular writer who has seen fit to include, as part of a disease description of diabetes, references to works by others writing in the field, is the author of P-4, a layman. This suggests that popular authors, for the most part, assume that what they have written is somehow 'sufficient unto itself'. Since the reader is not provided with the means whereby he or she may assess the work within the context of a critical tradition, the work may be said to be low in accountability.

[b]   The popular writer generally fails to delimit his claimed field of 'expertise'. Here the authorial assumption would appear to be that one individual (or a few together)[12] may possess sufficient medical knowledge to write an entire book of medical instruction. Moreover, as is apparent from Appendix D and Table 60, there appears to be little reticence on the part of popular authors to write numerous books of

medical instruction. In light of the current proliferation of knowledge in all aspects of medical science, a stance so strongly suggestive of medical omniscience must be seen as inconsistent with the principle of accountability.

[c]   As has been pointed out earlier, popular books less frequently use standarized biomedical terminology (p. 234) or numerical quantifications (p. 234). While the use of 'fuzzier' terminology (e.g. 'sugar' instead of 'glucose', or 'a lot of diabetics' instead of '75% of diabetics tested in study x') may appear to demystify the subject under discussion, this very lack of precision, unfortunately, diminishes the possibility that statements may be made in a manner sufficiently precise and nonambiguous so as to permit their being challenged by the readers in light of evidence published by other writers.

[d]   Finally, with respect to the distribution of sentences of pragmatic instruction (see Supplement A-2), popular books contained relatively more sentences of the imperious type than did textbooks (DD: 48% as compared to 39%–see Table 4). The higher distribution in popular books of this more 'verbally coercive' form of sentence is indicative of a more authoritarian approach to teaching, one which affords the reader no option with respect to carrying out the instruction.

In summary, the characteristic style of textbooks is formal and authoritative, and the characteristic style of popular books is informal and authoritarian.

c.   *Style as a function of differing assumptions concerning the author-reader relationship*

Stylistic differences between textbooks of medicine and popular home medical books may be seen as a function of differing authorial assumptions concerning the nature of the author-reader relationship.

In the case of textbooks, the relationship is one of 'master' to 'apprentice',[13] whereas in the case of popular books, the relationship may be described as that holding between a 'friendly consultant' and 'concerned client'.

Given the absence in all eight books of any editorial disclaimers to the effect that 'the views of the author(s) do not necessarily represent those of the editor(s)', it will be assumed that both the style and the contents of these books have, in each case, been 'underwritten', as it were, by the editor(s).[14]

Insofar as the editors of all three textbooks have each occupied highly prestigious positions in a number of hospitals and universities, have held membership in numerous professional societies, and have received numerous professional awards,[15] they, and the authors whose contributions they have approved, may be said to function as ideal-types of 'culture-bearers' for the medical establishment.[16] Thus, in the context of the 'master' role to which they have been assigned, they are expected not only to indoctrinate the 'apprentice-'reader with currently approved knowledge bearing upon medical theory and practice, but also, they are expected to do so in a style of language that is deemed 'fitting' to the social and intellectual assumptions of the members of the medical establishment which the 'apprentice'-reader (one assumes) aspires to join. Thus, the formality of language style may be seen as a powerful social cue to the reader that a physician of medicine is expected, at least in his professional communications with his peers, to assume a style of language that is systematic, coherent, precise, uniform, and impersonal.

Moreover, as was indicated earlier, textbook style is not only formal, but authoritative as well, that is, the editors and authors provide a number of indications that they are accountable[17] to the 'apprentice'-reader both for what they say as well as for how they say it. Thus the relationship holding between the physician-editors or authors, and the reader, is both reciprocal and binding: the 'apprentice' is expected to emulate the 'model' provided by the 'master',[18] and the 'master' in turn guarantees accountability with respect to accuracy, currency, comprehensiveness, and validity of argument. Hence, the 'master' may be legitimately challenged by the 'apprentice'-reader on any one of those accounts.[19]

By contrast, the relationship holding between popular author and reader, that of 'friendly consultant' to 'concerned client', is neither reciprocal nor binding. Under no directive to train 'apprentices', the popular author can circumvent the painstaking and time-consuming requirements of responsible scholarship; and under no constraint to provide a 'fitting' linguistic model for the reader, he is at liberty to use or to invent any number of colorful collo-quialisms[20] for the presentation of his material.

From the perspective of the reader, such colloquial 'markers' signal that there is little if any social or educational distance between the author and himself. It is proposed, however, that such markers may be seen as devices whereby the author tries to establish credibility and trust on the basis of an assumed 'friendship' with the reader, rather than on the basis of scientific discourse.[21] Furthermore, insofar as the author, through failure to use precise terminology, or to cite references to other works, precludes even the possibility of an informed 'debate' between himself and the reader, he may be accused of denying the reader the means of critical access to the material being presented. Thus, the popular author's ostensibly egalitarian and reassuring 'posture' of friendship paradoxically conceals an underlying 'stance' toward the reader which is not only authoritarian, but also, highly 'territorial' with respect to knowledge, a stance which is consistent with a low degree of accountability to the reader.[22]

A corresponding paradox manifests itself in textbooks, where the relationship between 'master'-author and 'apprentice'-reader is both impersonal and ostensibly nonegalitarian. However, all statements in textbooks, to the degree that they are statements of scientifically-formulated theories, or of scientifically validated facts, may be said to constitute the 'communal property' of all readers (all, that is, who have undergone the discipline of mastering the requisite background knowledge). Moreover, despite the alleged distance between the 'master'-author and the 'apprentice'-reader (a distance suggested by the formal style), the latter has both the means and the right (if not in fact the obligation) to challenge any of the author's statements that fail to meet the scientific criteria of accuracy, currency, comprehensiveness and validity of argument. Thus the nonegalitarian 'posture' of the textbook author paradoxically conceals an underlying egalitarian 'stance' which both assumes and guarantees the reader's right to equal access to, and participation in, scientific discourse. In summary, the formal and authoritative style of textbooks is consistent with a high degree of accountability to the reader.

NOTES

1. For a definition of 'nondiscursive elements', see Part Two, I: 5.
2. Some of these differences will be cited again in relation to distinguishing the respective styles of textbooks and popular books.
3. The initials 'DD' will be placed before all figures whose statistical source was the Disease Descriptions.
4. The initials 'SH' will be placed before all figures whose statistical source was the Selected Headings.
5. An asterisk placed after each numbered table indicates that a companion graph appears on the page following that table.
6. This finding was contrary to the expectation of the writer.
7. As before, the initials 'DD' will precede all figures whose statistical source was the Disease Descriptions, and the initials 'SH' will precede all figures whose statistical source was the Selected Headings.
8. Martin Joos, in *The Five Clocks* (Bloomington, 1962), identifies five different 'clocks', or styles of English: intimate, casual, consultative, formal, and frozen. The style of textbook discourse most closely resembles his 'formal' style: 'Formal style is designed to inform . . . (it) is strictly determined by the absence of participation. (The speaker) may speak as if he were not present, avoiding such allusions to his own existence as "I", "me", "mine", with the possible exception of "one" . . .
    Lacking all personal support, the text must fight its own battles . . . Robbed of personal links to reality, . . . it endeavours to employ only logical links . . . Back-

ground information is woven into the text in complex sentences. Exempt from interruption, the text organizes itself into paragraphs: the paragraphs are linked explicitly . . . The defining features of formal style are two: (1) Detachment and (2) Cohesion' (Joos 1962: 25-26).

9. Numerical quantifications include Afabic numerals, percentages, etc. However, quantifications which were expressed in words (e.g. 'five percent') were not included in the calculations.

10. With respect to the notion of a 'critical tradition', the reader has previously been referred to the works of Karl Popper.

11. Such criticisms appearing in medical journals may also play a role in helping professors of medicine make informed decisions concerning which textbooks they will recommend to their students for the subsequent academic term.

12. Two of the five popular books are single-authored. The remainder have, respectively, two, six, and 31 authors. In contrast, the average number of contributors per textbook is 160 (see Table 19).

13. I am grateful to Irwin Gopnick for having suggested this distinction to me.

14. In the case of P-2 and P-5, the author and editor are one and the same person.

15. See Appendix C.

16. In Part Two, II: 3, it has been shown (1) that the introductory discourses of all three textbooks contain references to respected predecessors, and (2) that all textbook dedications are addressed to coprofessionals. This would seem to confirm that textbook editors are highly conscious of their roles as 'culture-bearers'.

17. With respect to a closely related notion, namely, that of responsibility, Joos (1962), makes the following provocative observations: 'The community's survival depends on cooperation; and adequate cooperation depends on recognizing the more and the less responsible types of persons around us. We need to identify the natural burden-bearers of the community so that we can give them the responsibility which is heaviest of all: we make them responsible for cooperation itself. Then the majority of us can function carefree in our square and round niches, free of the burden of maintaining the cooperation-net which joins us all . . . . Responsible language does not palter. It is explicit. It commits the speaker. The responsible speaker is under a sort of almost morbid compulsion to leave himself no way out of his commitment. The responsibility-dialect does not mumble; its grammar does not contradict itself; its semantics doesn't weasle. . .' (p. 15).

18. The implied instruction is two-fold: 'Consider what I say, and say it as I say'. The extent to which the 'apprentice' has succeeded is subsequently determined through the examination process.

19. The physician who reviews textbooks in medical journals may be seen as an 'ideal' reader-critic. But of course any reader can provide critical 'feedback', whether directly (via a letter to the textbook editor), or indirectly (via a letter or article submitted to a medical journal).

20. See Supplement A-3.

21. In relation to this issue,.it may be seen that the properties of 'casual' style (described in Joos (1962: 19) closely approximate many of the stylistic properties of popular books: 'Casual style is for friends, acquaintances, insiders; addressed to a stranger, it serves to make him an insider simply by treating him as an insider. Negatively, there is absence of background information and no reliance on listeners' participation . . . it pays the addressee the compliment of supposing that he will understand without those aids. On the positive side, we have two devices which do

the same job directly: (1) ellipsis, and (2) slang, the two defining features of casual style'.

22. This paradox manifests itself not only in books of medical instruction, but throughout the broad spectrum of medical interactions in society; whenever, in fact, authoritarian sources of reassurance are favored over authoritative sources of scientifically-based medical knowledge. In Supplement A-4, discursive samples from the Texts have been provided to show that popular books in general are far more reassuring and optimistic than are textbooks.

Differences in Contents

1. DIFFERENCES IN SCOPE

The scope of each book of medical instruction has been investigated from two perspectives: (a) broad and (b) narrow.

a. The broad scope, i.e. the numbers and types of topics addressed by an entire book, has been determined from an examination of its Selected Headings.

b. The narrow scope, i.e. the numbers and types of key concepts in terms of which a specified portion of a book is explained (in the case of this study, a Disease Description of diabetes mellitus), has been determined from an examination of its Schema (i.e. the set of bold-type headings typically interspersed throughout each Disease Description).

The broad scope

The reader will recall that, in order to cross-compare the broad scopes of all books, the Selected Headings of each book were respectively 'mapped' on to an external standard, the 'List of Three-digit Categories' (see Supplement B-1(a). The results of this comparison are as follows.

1. Respectively 82%, 76% and 82% of the 17 'Categories' in the 'List of Three-digit Categories' were 'covered' by the Selected Headings of T-1, T-2, and T-3 respectively, yielding a textbook average of 80% (see Table 39 and its Graph [a]).

2. Respectively 94%, 53%, 88%, 94%, and 82% of the 17 'Categories' in the 'List' were 'covered' by the Selected Headings of P-1, P-2, P-3, P-4, and P-5 respectively, yielding a popular average of 82% (see Table 39 and its Graph [a]).

Therefore, since popular books as a group 'covered' 2% more[1] of the 'Categories' on the 'List of Three-digit Categories' than did textbooks as a group, the broad scope of popular books was shown to be slightly greater than that of textbooks.

3. With respect to Selected Headings which were left over after the mapping procedure (see Supplement B-1 [b]), the following conclusions apply:

Textbooks. Each of the three textbooks contained a heading referring to an introductory section in which basic principles pertaining to the doctor-patient relationship were set forth: in T-1, 'The Physician and the Patient', in T-2, 'The Nature of Medicine', and in T-3, 'The Approach to the Patient'. Other headings which were left over in textbooks may be seen as possible indicators of emerging topics or 'specialties' in medicine, for example, in T-2, 'Granulomatous Diseases of Unproved Etiology', and in T-3, 'Diseases of Medical Management', 'Medical Problems Associated with Alcoholism', and 'Adolescent Medicine'.

Popular Books. The reader will note that most of the Selected Headings which were left over in popular books reflect the general tendency of popular books to include discourse pertaining to sexual, social, and occupational factors relating to health and disease.

4. With respect to 'Categories' from the 'List' which were unmapped (see Supplement B-1 [c]), the least frequently mapped 'Categories' were the following: 'XI: Complications of Pregnancy, Childbirth, and the Puerperium', and 'XV: Certain Conditions Originating in the Perinatal Period'. Thus, medical problems pertaining to a relatively large proportion of the population, i.e. pregnant women and newborns, are relatively ignored in both groups of the selected books.

5. Supplement B-1(c) also indicates that the following 'Categories' are universally addressed in all of the eight selected books:

'III: Endocrine, Nutritional, and Metabolic Diseases, and Immunity Disorders'
'V: Mental Disorders'
'VII: Diseases of the Circulatory System'
'VIII: Diseases of the Respiratory System'
'IX: Diseases of the Digestive System'
'XIII: Diseases of the Musculoskeletal System and Connective Tissue'
'XVII: Injury and Poisoning'

The narrow scope

The reader will recall that in order to cross-compare the narrow scopes of all Disease Descriptions, the Schema of each Description was 'mapped' into the set of 32 chapter headings of *Joslin's* (see Table 29).

Table 29 clearly indicates that the Schemata of textbooks correlate far more closely with the 32 chapter headings of *Joslin's* than do the Schemata of popular books. This difference may be expressed mathematically: out of a possible 96 correlations[2] in the case of textbooks, 58 (i.e. 60%) were a-chieved. By contrast, out of a possible 160 correlations[3] in the case of popular books, only 21 (i.e. 13%) were achieved. Thus, bold-type headings from text-book Schemata could be correlated almost five times more frequently with *Joslin's* headings than could the bold-type headings from popular Schemata. Moreover, there were only 7 *Joslin's* headings to which no textbook heading could be correlated, as compared to 18 *Joslin's* headings to which no popular heading could be correlated.

It is interesting to note that neither textbook nor popular Schemata con-tained headings corresponding to *Joslin's* Nos. 29 and 30 (respectively, 'Emotional Factors in Diabetes' and 'Socioeconomic Considerations in the Life of a Diabetic').

Other differences revealed in Table 29 are likely to be of more interest to the diabetologist than to the general reader.

In summary, while it has been demonstrated that the broad scope of popular books is slightly greater than that of textbooks (82% in popular books as compared to 80% in textbooks), it has also been demonstrated that the narrow scope in textbooks is greater than that of popular books (60% as compared to 13%). Thus while textbooks as compared to popular books may restrict the number of topics which they address, a specific topic (i.e. 'dia-betes mellitus') is elaborated more fully, that is to say, it is described in terms of more concepts than is the case in popular books.

2.   DIFFERENCES IN THE PORTRAYAL OF *HOMO MEDICABILIS*

The following conclusions are based upon data[4] appearing in Part Two in the form of numbered tables, graphs, and supplements. Since each numbered table in Part Two has an identically numbered companion graph immediately following it, only the tables will be referred to below. An asterisk will be placed after the number of each table cited below to remind the reader of this fact. Also, with respect to the numbered supplements, the reader is encouraged to refer to them when indicated, as they contain either explana-tions or exemplifications of the various classes of terms which will be dealt with below.

a.   *Homo medicabilis* Type P

With respect to portrayals of *homo medicabilis,* the following set of conclusions applies to popular home medical books as a group:

I.   Popular books describe *homo medicabilis* as a body endowed with a mind.

This conclusion is supported by the following facts:

1.   The term 'body' (see Supplement B-14) has a relatively higher distribution in popular books than in textbooks (DD: 0.2% as compared to 0.03% —see Table 12*, and SH: 1% as compared to 0%—see Table 51*).

2.   Terms belonging to the domains of psychiatry, neurology, and behavioral psychology (see Supplement B-17) have a relatively higher distribution in popular books than in textbooks (SH: 8% as compared to 3%—see Table 54*). Supplement B-17 also shows that the terms 'mental' and 'mind' are found exclusively in Selected Headings of popular books.

II.   Popular books describe the body both in terms of its external as well as internal parts.

This conclusion is supported by the fact that nouns which name anatomical structures of the human organism (see Supplement B-16) have a relatively higher distribution in popular books than in textbooks (SH: 13% as compared to 8%—see Table 53*). Also, with respect to this set of nouns, popular books contain a higher percentage of nouns naming 'overt' anatomical structures than do textbooks (SH: 49% as compared to 7%—see Table 53*).

III.   *Homo medicabilis* is less often described as a 'patient' than as a 'person', and is clearly located within the context of an ongoing family and social life.

This conclusion is supported by the following facts:

1.   With respect to all nouns referring to human subjects, popular books contain relatively fewer Type A nouns[5] than textbooks (DD: 37% as compared to 71%—see Table 13*). With respect to Type B nouns,[6] it was found that popular books contain relatively more of both Type B_1 nouns and Type B_2 nouns[7] than do textbooks (DD: 83% as compared to 23%—see Table 14*).

2.   With respect to terms naming certain sexual, social, and developmental states or roles of the human organism (see Supplement B-18), it was found that popular books contain a relatively higher distribution than textbooks (SH: 6% as compared to 1%—see Table 55*).

IV.   Although popular books (1) clearly acknowledge the existence of specific diseases, they (2) assume that the given state of *homo medicabilis* is that of health rather than disease, and that disease is preventable.

These conclusions are supported by the following facts:

1. With respect to terms for aberrant states and for indicators of aberrant states (see Supplement B-11), it was found that popular books contain a relatively higher distribution of Type Two terms[8] than do textbooks (SH: 21% as compared to 1%—see Table 48*). Therefore, popular books clearly acknowledge the existence of specific diseases.

2. With respect to the terms 'health', 'prevention', and their variants (see Supplement B-13), it was found that popular books contain a relatively higher distribution than do textbooks (DD: 0.1% as compared to 0.01%—see Table 11*, and SH: 2% as compared to 0%—see Table 50*).

V. Disease manifests itself in symptoms for which relief is available.

This conclusion is supported by the following facts:

1. With respect to specific terms for indicators of aberrant states (i.e. Type Two terms), it may be noted that popular books contain far more terms referring to specific symptoms and signs than do textbooks (SH: see Supplement B-11).

2. With respect to terms belonging to the domain of treatment or care of the human organism (see Supplement B-12), it was found that popular books contain a relatively higher distribution than do textbooks (SH: 7% as compared to 1%—see Table 49*).

VI. Measures pertaining to the prevention of disease, or to the relief of its symptoms, are accessible to the reader through such 'natural' means as diet, dietary supplements, massage, rest, and exercise.

This conclusion is supported by the fact that popular books have a relatively higher distribution of terms which name so-called 'natural' approaches to the maintenance of health (see Supplement B-19), than do textbooks (DD: 2.4% as compared to 0.6%—see Table 9* and SH: 4% as compared to 1%—see Table 56*).

VII. Insofar as the concepts of 'health' and 'prevention' are emphasized (Conclusion IV), and insofar as disease is said to manifest itself in symptoms and signs for which relief is available (Conclusion V), and insofar as both the prevention of disease or relief of its symptoms are claimed to be accessible through certain 'natural' approaches (Conclusion VI), it may be concluded that popular home medical books not only present a relatively more optimistic outlook[9] than textbooks, but that, moreover, they assign a greater degree of autonomy to *homo medicabilis* with respect to the 'government' of his own biological state.

b.   *Homo medicabilis* Type T

With respect to the manner in which *homo medicabilis* is described in textbooks, the following set of conclusions applies:

I.   Textbooks of medicine describe *homo medicabilis* as a biological system
with constituent subsystems.
     This conclusion is supported by the fact that the term 'system' or its
variants (see Supplement B-15) has a relatively higher distribution in textbooks than in popular books (SH: 6% as compared to 2%—see Table 52*).
Moreover, whereas textbooks name eight different kinds of systems, popular
books name only six (see Supplement B-15[c]).

II.   The functions and malfunctions of this system are accounted for largely
in terms of measurable alterations of biochemical values.
     This conclusion is supported by the fact that terms naming biochemicals
are relatively more numerous in textbooks than in popular books (DD: 4.5%
as compared to 2.6%—see Table 8*). Moreover, textbooks contain a relatively
higher distribution of quantifications expressed in Arabic numerals than do
popular books (DD: 1.3% as compared to 0.4%—see Table 15*). The greater
prevalence in textbooks of terms naming biochemicals is also evident when
one compares the terminology found in the Schemata of textbook Disease
Descriptions (see Tables 21 to 23) with the Schemata of popular Disease
Descriptions (Tables 24 to 28). For external confirmation of this general
trend in textbook vs popular literature, the reader may also refer to Appendix
F, 'Key Headings in Two Books Devoted to the Topic of Diabetes Mellitus'.

III.   Textbooks assume that the various subsystems, structures, and functions
of the system are highly predisposed toward such aberrant states as diseases
and disorders.
     This conclusion is supported by the following evidence:
     1.   With respect to terms referring to human subjects, Type A,[10] text-
books show a relatively higher distribution than do popular books (DD: 71%
as compared to 37%—see Table 13*).
     2.   With respect to terms referring to aberrant states, Type One,[11] the
reader will note that in textbooks these terms are more frequently applied to
subsystems, structures, and functions than they are in popular books (DD:
Supplement B-8).

IV.   Textbooks assume that the appropriate method of diagnosing and correcting such states involves carefully-measured biochemical agents, the

administration and use of which are to be carried out under the close external supervision and control of a licensed medical doctor.

This statement is supported by the following arguments:

1.   As has already been noted, terms naming biochemicals, and quantifications expressed in Arabic numerals, are relatively more numerous in textbooks than in popular books (see Conclusion I).

2.   In textbooks in particular, terms naming biochemicals were found to contain a large subset of terms naming pharamacological agents, i.e. either 'generic' or 'brand' names of drugs. Most of these terms were preceded by quantifications expressed in Arabic numerals, and found in contexts dealing with therapy. Since, by law, the administration of many such drugs requires that one be a licensed physician, the layman will not have legal access to them. Furthermore, even were he to gain access to them illegally, he would not ordinarily possess sufficient background knowledge (either in human biochemistry or pharmacology) to be able to administer them with accuracy and safety. The textbook author, then, obviously assumes that the reader has both legal access to, as well as sufficient knowlege about, the pharmacological agents which are recommended for diagnostic or therapeutic use.

In summary, then, to the degree that textbooks account for aberrant states largely in terms of measurable alterations of biochemical values, and infer from this that the proper correction of such aberrant states demands the administration of measured pharmacological agents, and insofar as only physicians may legally administer most of these agents, it follows that textbook authors assume that physicians should be mainly responsible for the supervision and control of aberrant states in others. Therefore, textbooks assign less autonomy to *homo medicabilis* with respect to the 'government' of his own biological state than do popular books.

V.   Therefore, insofar as the selected textbooks (a) emphasize that the biological system is highly predisposed to aberrant states (Conclusion III), (b) fail to emphasize, as do popular books, the notions of 'health' or 'prevention', or to underline certain so-called 'natural' approaches to the maintenance of health, and (c) give priority to the role of the physician rather than the patient with respect to the control of the patient's aberrant states (Conclusion IV), we may conclude that textbooks present a less optimistic view,[12] and that they assign *homo medicabilis* less autonomy, than do the popular books of medical instruction.

Finally, although popular books may provide their readers with general instructions in health care, and with reassurance in alleviating their anxieties, nevertheless it should be stated that insofar as these books are authoritarian and are frequently written in an emotive style, the reader may be at risk in misinterpreting the discourse. This state of affairs might well occur should the reader, lacking sufficient background knowledge, conclude, on the basis of what the writer has written, either that a disorder is present when it is not, or (more seriously perhaps), erroneously judge that certain of his signs or symptoms are so innocuous as not to require the attention of a physician.

NOTES

1. This percentage would have been greater still except for the fact that the Selected Headings of P-2 'covered' only 53% of the 'Categories', hence considerably lowered the popular average (see Table 39).
2. This figure was arrived at by multiplying the number of *Joslin's* headings (32) by the number of textbook Schemata (3).
3. This figure was arrived at by multiplying the number of *Joslin's* headings (32) by the number of popular Schemata (5).
4. All figures preceded by the initials 'DD' indicate that the statistical source of the data is the Disease Descriptions. Figures preceded by the initials 'SH' indicate that the statistical source of the data is the Selected Headings.
5. Type A nouns contain the semantic component 'one who is sick'. Examples are: 'patient', 'diabetic', etc.
6. Type B nouns constitute the remaining subset of all nouns referring to human subjects.
7. Type B_1 nouns are nouns which name certain 'biosocial' roles, such as those defined by age (e.g. 'child'), sex (e.g. 'woman'), family membership (e.g. 'parent') and occupation (e.g. 'housewife'). Type B_2 nouns include the nouns 'person(s)' and 'people'.
8. Examples of Type One terms for aberrant states are the terms 'disease', 'disorder', etc. Type One terms for indicators of aberrant states include the terms 'symptom', 'sign', 'manifestation', etc. Type One terms, then, are *general* terms.

   Examples of Type Two terms for aberrant states are: 'diabetes', 'myocardial infarction', 'Cushing's syndrome', and so on. Type Two terms for indicators of aberrant states include: 'insomnia', 'headache', 'cough', and so on. Type Two terms, then, are *specific* terms.

   Given that the Selected Headings constitute, for the most part, the first 'level' of the classification of the contents of the selected books, it is interesting to note that in textbooks, Type Two terms exist either at the second, third, or fourth 'level' of classification, rather than at the first 'level' (as in the popular books). It is obvious, then, that textbooks organize disease according to much higher levels of abstraction.
9. See also Supplement A-4, in which appear sentences which offer reassurance, encouragement, and hope to the popular reader.
10. Type A terms contain the semantic component 'one who is sick'. Examples are: 'patient' and 'diabetic'.
11. As indicated earlier, Type One terms name general classes of aberrant states (e.g. 'disease' and 'disorder') and general classes of indicators of aberrant states (e.g. 'symptom', 'sign', and 'manifestation').
12. See p. 258, paragraph 3.

PART FOUR

Appendices and Bibliography

'Genealogies' of Books of Medical Instruction

GENEALOGY OF T-1

1. Harrison, Tinsley Randolph, ed. *Principles of Internal Medicine.* Ed.-in-chief T.R. Harrison. Eds. P.B. Beeson, W.H. Resnik, G.W. Thorn, M.M. Wintrobe. Philadelphia: Blakiston, 1950.
   1590 pp., illus., pl., diags., ch., tab., 27 cm.
   Contains bibliography throughout text.
2. Harrison, Tinsley Randolph, ed. *Principles of Internal Medicine.* 2nd ed. Eds. T.R. Harrison (and others). London: Lewis, 1954.
   1703 pp., illus., 26.5 cm.
   Bibliography.
3. Harrison, Tinsley Randolph, ed. *Principles of Internal Medicine.* 3rd ed. Eds. T.R. Harrison (and others). New York: McGraw-Hill, 1958.
   1782 pp., illus., 25.5 cm.
   Bibliography.
4. Harrison, Tinsely Randolph, ed. *Principles of Internal Medicine.* 4th ed. Eds. T.R. Harrison (and others). New York: McGraw-Hill, 1962.
   1947 pp., illus., 26 cm.
5. Harrison, Tinsley Randolph, ed. *Principles of Internal Medicine.* 5th ed. Eds. T.R. Harrison (and others). New York: McGraw-Hill, c.1966.
   2 vols., 26 cm.
6. *Harrison's Principles of Internal Medicine.* 6th ed. Eds. Maxwell M. Wintrobe (et. al.). New York: Blakiston, 1970.
   2106 pp., illus.
7. *Principles of Internal Medicine.* 7th ed. Eds. Maxwell M. Wintrobe (et. al.). New York: McGraw-Hill, c.1974.
   2044, 8, 179 pp., illus., plates.
8. *Harrison's Principles of Internal Medicine.* 8th ed. Eds. George W. Thorn (et. al.). New York: McGraw-Hill, c.1977.
   2088, 108 pp., illus.

GENEALOGY OF T-2

1. Cecil, Russell LaFayette, ed. *Textbook of Medicine by American Authors*. Philadelphia: Saunders, 1928.
2. Cecil, Russell LaFayette, ed. *Textbook of Medicine by American Authors*. 2nd ed. rev. and entirely reset. Philadelphia: Saunders, 1930.
3. Cecil, Russell LaFayette, ed. *Textbook of Medicine by American Authors*. 3rd ed. rev. and entirely reset. Philadelphia: Saunders, 1934.
4. Cecil, Russell LaFayette, ed. *Textbook of Medicine by American Authors*. 4th ed. rev. and entirely reset. Philadelphia: Saunders, 1938.
5. Cecil, Russell LaFayette, ed. *Textbook of Medicine by American Authors*. 5th ed. rev. and entirely reset. Philadelphia: Saunders, 1940.
   Cecil, Russell LaFayette, ed. *Textbook of Medicine. Supplement: Treatment of Infections with Penicillin*. By D.G. Anderson and C.S. Keefer. Philadelphia: Saunders, 1944.
6. Cecil, Russell LaFayette, ed. *Textbook of Medicine by American Authors*. 6th ed. rev. and entirely reset. Philadelphia: Saunders, 1943.
   1566 pp., front, illus., pl. (diag.), map. diags., ch., tab.
   Contains bibliography throughout text.
7. Cecil, Russell LaFayette, ed. *Textbook of Medicine*. 7th ed. Philadelphia: Saunders, 1947.
   1730 pp., illus., pl., map, diags., ch., tab.
8. Cecil, Russell LaFayette, ed. *Textbook of Medicine*. 8th ed. Ed. by R.L. Cecil, R.F. Loeb; Assoc. eds., A.B. Gutman, Walsh McDermott, H.G. Wolff. Philadelphia: Saunders, 1951.
   1627 pp., illus., maps, ch., tab., 26 cm.
   Contains bibliography throughout text.
9. Cecil, Russell LaFayette, ed. *Textbook of Medicine*. 9th ed. Ed. by R. L. Cecil, R.F. Loeb; Assoc. eds. A.B. Gutman (et. al.). Philadelphia: Saunders, 1955.
   1786 pp., illus., pl., map, diags., ch., tab., 26 cm.
   Bibliography.
10. Cecil, Russell LaFayette, ed. *Textbook of Medicine*. 10th ed. Ed. by R.L. Cecil, R.F. Loeb. Philadelphia: Saunders, 1959.
    1665, lxxxix pp., illus., 26 cm.
    References.

11. Cecil, Russell, LaFayette, ed. (Cecil-Loeb) *Textbook of Medicine.* 11th ed. Ed. by P.B. Beeson and W. McDermott; Assoc. eds. A.G. Bearn (et. al.). Philadelphia: Saunders, 1963.
    2 vols., illus., 26.5 cm.
12. Cecil, Russell LaFayette. *Cecil-Loeb Textbook of Medicine.* 12th ed. Ed. by Paul B. Beeson and Walsh McDermott. Philadelphia: Saunders, c.1967.
    2 vols., illus., 26 cm.
13. Cecil, Russell LaFayette, ed. *Cecil-Loeb Textbook of Medicine.* 13th ed. Ed. by Paul B. Beeson and Walsh McDermott. Philadelphia: Saunders, 1971.
    2 vols., illus., 27 cm., 1923, LI p.
14. Beeson, Paul and Walsh McDermott. *Textbook of Medicine.* 14th ed. Philadelphia: Saunders, 1975.
    1864, (78) pp., illus.

GENEALOGY OF T-3

1. Osler (Sir) William Bart. *Principles and Practice of Medicine, Designed for the Use of Practitioners and Students of Medicine.* New York: Appleton, 1892.
   1079 pp.
2. Osler (Sir) William Bart. *Principles and Practice of Medicine, Designed for the Use of Practitioners and Students of Medicine.* 2nd ed. New York: Appleton, 1895.
   1143 pp.
3. Osler (Sir) William Bart. *Principles and Practice of Medicine, Designed for the Use of Practitioners and Students of Medicine.* 3rd ed. New York: Appleton, 1898.
   1181 pp.
4. Osler (Sir) William Bart. *Principles and Practice of Medicine, Designed for the Use of Practitioners and Students of Medicine.* 4th ed. New York: Appleton, 1901.
   1182 pp.
5. Osler (Sir) William Bart. *Principles and Practice of Medicine, Designed for the Use of Practitioners and Students of Medicine.* 5th ed. New York: Appleton, 1903.
   1182 pp.
6. Osler (Sir) William Bart. *Principles and Practice of Medicine, Designed for the Use of Practitioners and Students of Medicine.* 6th ed.

Thoroughly rev. New York: Appleton, 1905.
1143 pp.

7. Osler (Sir) William Bart. *Principles and Practice of Medicine, Designed for the Use of Practitioners and Students of Medicine.* 7th ed. Thoroughly rev. New York: Appleton, 1909.
1143 pp.

8. Osler (Sir) William Bart. *Principles and Practice of Medicine, Designed for the Use of Practitioners and Students of Medicine.* 8th ed. Largely re-written and thoroughly rev. with the assistance of Thomas McCrae. New York: Appleton, 1912.
1225 pp., illus.

9. Osler (Sir) William Bart. *Principles and Practice of Medicine, Designed for the Use of Practitioners and Students of Medicine.* 9th ed. Thoroughly rev. by the late Sir William Bart Osler, and Thomas McCrae. New York: Appleton, 1923.
1168 pp.

10. Osler (Sir) William Bart. *Principles and Practice of Medicine, Designed for the Use of Practitioners and Students of Medicine.* 10th ed. Thoroughly rev. by T. McCrae. New York: Appleton (c.1925).
1223 pp., illus., 24 cm.

11. Osler (Sir) William Bart. *Principles and Practice of Medicine, Designed for the Use of Practitioners and Students of Medicine.* 11th ed. Rev. by Thomas McCrae. New York: Appleton, 1930.
1237 pp., diags., ch., O.

12. Osler (Sir) William Bart. *Principles and Practice of Medicine, Designed for the Use of Practitioners and Students of Medicine.* 12th ed. Rev. by Thomas McCrae. New York: Appleton-Century (c.1935).
1196 pp., illus., diags., ch., tab., O.

13. Osler (Sir) William Bart. *Principles and Practice of Medicine, Designed for the Use of Practitioners and Students of Medicine.* 13th ed. Rev. by H.A. Christian. New York: Appleton-Century, c.1938.
1424 pp., illus., diags., tab., O.

14. *Principles and Practice of Medicine.* 14th semicentennial (1892-1942) ed. Originally written by the late Sir William Osler, Designed for the Use of Practitioners and Students of Medicine. By H.A. Christian. New York: Appleton-Century, c.1942).
1475 pp., illus., diags., tab., O.
Contains bibliography throughout text.

15. *Principles and Practice of Medicine.* 15th ed. Originally written by the late Sir William Osler, Designed for the Use of Practitioners and Students of Medicine. By H.A. Christian. New York: Appleton-

Century, c.1944.
1498 pp., illus., diags., tab., O.
Contains bibliography throughout text.

16. Christian, Henry Asbury. *Principles and Practice of Medicine,* 16th ed. Originally Written by William Osler, Designed for the Use of Practitioners and Students of Medicine. New York: Appleton-Century, c.1947.
1539 pp., illus., tab., 24 cm.
Contains bibliography throughout text.

17. *The Principles and Practice of Medicine,* ed. by A.M. Harvey (et. al.). 17th ed. New York: Appleton, c.1968.
1472 pp., illus.
Originally written by W. Osler.
Previous ed. by H.A. Christian.

18. *The Principles and Practice of Medicine.* 18th ed. Ed. by A. McGehee Harvey (et. al.). New York: Appleton-Century-Crofts, c.1972.
1650 pp., illus.
Originally written by W. Osler.

19. *The Principles and Practice of Medicine.* 19th ed. Ed. by A. McGehee Harvey (et. al.). New York: Appleton-Century-Crofts, c.1976.
1892 pp., illus.

GENEALOGY OF P-5

1. Fishbein, Morris. *Good Housekeeping's Pocket Medical Encyclopedia.* New York: Hearst Corp., c.1956.
2. Fishbein, Morris. *The Handy Home Medical Adviser.*[1] c.1952.
3. Fishbein, Morris. *The Handy Home Medical Adviser and Concise Medical Encyclopedia.* c.1957. Rev. ed. 1963, Rev. ed. 1973.

NOTE

1. The 'genealogy' of P-5 has been confined to editions which bear in their titles the phrase 'The Handy Home Medical Adviser'. Although there have been numerous editions (10) of a book bearing the phrase 'Modern Home Medical Adviser' (published between 1935 and 1961), these editions may not, strictly speaking, be cited as part of the 'genealogy' of P-5.

Critical Reviews of Books of Medical Instruction

REVIEW OF T-1
from *Annuals of Internal Medicine* (1977), Vol. 87, pp. 128-129.

The eighth edition of 'Harrison' maintains the standards that we have the right to associate with a textbook that has survived for 27 years and that has been translated into eight languages. It is true that popularity does not equate with excellence and, indeed, the first edition was considered to be an unconventional book. It attempted a unified approach by presenting the *principles* of internal medicine. The editors stated that a textbook of medicine should recapitulate the steps and the processes of thinking by which a physician reaches a diagnosis—verily a 'problem-solving' approach, years in advance of the popularity of that overworked term.

The *Annals* reviewer of the first edition was enthusiastic about the new approach and the content related to it. He was less enthusiastic about the 'bread and butter' disease description portion, considering it no better than most available textbooks and inferior to many. My analysis of subsequent editions indicates that most of the revision has taken place in this area, with felicitous results. Another curmudgeon-like criticism was that the two volumes of the book weighted an unwieldy eight and one-half pounds. I am now glad to state that, even if the contributors have quadrupled in number, the current weight of the single volume is a manageable six pounds and two ounces! It still might be more manageable in the slightly more expensive, albeit heavier, two-volume edition.

What has been done to improve this edition? The reader will find that there are major revisions. Sections on hematology and cerebrovascular disease have been rewritten. New chapters have been added, notably on the adult respiratory distress syndrome, host-defense mechanisms, emergencies in medicine, fertility control, sexual counselling and a depressing but realistic chapter on aging, involution, and senescence. I would have preferred a little comfort as far as the latter is concerned with some emphasis on psychic potential rather than somatic deterioration. The technological imperative has been maintained by the addition of new information on echocardiography and computerized axial tomography. The indications for and capabilities of fiber optic bronchoscopy and endoscopy have been updated.

What further needs to be done to improve this textbook? I must restate that it is impossible to go into a detailed recitation of peccadilloes of content and I believe that the editors and authors are unlikely to be men of casual attitude to fact. To paraphrase David Hume, any point of medicine that is so obvious that it scarcely admits of dispute, but at the same time so important that it cannot be too often inculcated, requires some method of handling, and the classical textbook of this kind seems as good a way as any. However, there are various areas of emphasis that may irritate. Since this is also a reference textbook one cannot call for undue simplicity or argue with four pages on carcinoid disease and eight pages on virtually untreatable genetic disorders of supporting tissue. However, if such information is included for the sake of completeness, why not also include mundane and frustrating topics of prevention, such as how to control smoking (which gets 10 lines) or alter the eating habits of patients with hyperlipidemia. Why not discuss in greater depth stroke and post-myocardial-infarction rehabilitation, the care of the dying patient, the special problems of the geriatric patient, or the value of the annual physical examination. Do not these areas require equal time?

It is hard to review this type of textbook since it has to be so many things to so many people, and it will not satisfy all. Most who buy it will undoubted obtain value for their money. I am still concerned about the unwieldiness of all the information included, but the solution presently escapes me. Computers appeal but somehow constitute the barren triumph of science over reason. Possibly there should be a system of starring or color coding to guide the reader along the 'track' that he most requires. There might even be a symbol that means 'worth a detour'! (Thomas C. Gibson, M.D., M.R.C.P., University of Vermont, Department of Medicine, Burlington, Vermont)

REVIEW OF T-2
from *Dermatology* (Nov. 1976), p. 702.

The fourteenth edition of this long-time standard textbook of medicine is a fitting tribute to Cecil and Loeb, who were the original editors of this book. The contributors to this edition constitute the 'Who's Who' of medicine and its specialties. For the dermatologist this is a basic, and surprisingly inexpensive, two-volume compilation not only for the extensive discussion of dermatoses, but especially for the many internal disorders which may show cutaneous manifestations.

Herman Beerman, M.D.,
Philadelphia, PA.

REVIEW OF T-2
from *Delaware Medical Journal* (May 1976), Vol. 48, No. 1, p. 302.

The 14th edition of this classic tome is similar in size to the 13th published four years ago. It has approximately the same number of pages: 1970 compared to 1974, and 67 lines per page to the old edition's 65 lines.

The authors have made a few changes in organization and have updated content. They have tried to make a major emphasis on therapy. The sections on genetics, environment, and nutrition in particular have been enlarged.

Three mistakes in the copy have been made, but the authors and publishers are making drastic efforts to correct them. Anyone not receiving these corrections can get them by contacting the publishers.

This book continues to be one of the major texts in the field of Internal Medicine—many is the person who has wished he had all the information stored in his memory that is packed into these pages. As a major text it demands space in every reference library, and it is preferred by some students over the other texts because of its easy readability and manner of organization.

REVIEW OF T-2
from *Plastic and Reconstructive Surgery* (Oct. 1976), p. 498.

Although familiar with the work, it is nearly impossible for a surgeon to write an adequate review of Beeson and McDermott's Fourteenth Edition of *Textbook of Medicine*. It is an encyclopedic compendium of virtually every affliction of human beings, and it probably contains more useful information than any other single volume in the medical literature.

The unique subject numbering system simulates the flavor of the Merck Manual, yet it provides the reader with an excellent classification of knowledge which can be located expediently. Exceptions to this style are the superb first four chapters by Beeson, Feinstein, Myers, and McDermott on the Nature of Medicine. These chapters, and an excellent chapter on the Use and Interpretation of Laboratory Derived Data (by Wyngaarden), have been written in a more easy-to-read prose than the organ system sections. The above general chapters contain valuable thoughts on and philosophical approaches to human biology, ones which will be valuable to all practitioners of medicine and surgery. Part II covers genetic principles, Part IV the immune diseases, Part V the connective tissues, and Part XX the cutaneous diseases with their systemic manifestations. The last will be of special interest to plastic surgeons.

The earlier editions of this *Textbook of Medicine,* edited by Dr. Loeb (or still earlier by Dr. Cecil), were directed particularly to the needs of medical students. However, this Fourteenth Edition appears to be edited more for use by practicing physicians and surgeons. Plastic surgeons will find the volume most beneficial in providing the background information needed to converse intelligently with medical consultants. The work can only be described as an outstanding source of reference material for surgeons, one containing much seldom needed information about all types of human disease. It is so complete that the present volume suffers somewhat from the small print, the less than adequate illustrations, and too few references. However, if purchased and used even occasionally, this book can do much to prevent the retreat from basic human biology to which the surgical specialist succumbs without realizing what is happening. That is only one of the rewards for owning a volume such as *Textbook of Medicine,* which contains contributions from many of the great internists of our time.

Erle E. Peacock, Jr., M.D.

REVIEW OF T-2
from *Unlisted Drugs* (July 1976), Vol. 28, No. 7, p. 124.

An American classic, the 'Beeson and McDermott' is a direct successor of 'Cecil' (and 'Loeb') the original multiauthor textbook of medicine, on which generations of US (and many other) medical students grew since the 1920s. The fourteenth edition is slightly larger than the thirteenth, although it has actually less pages due to judicious use of typeface and typographic margins; in general, the typographic presentation is superlative as is evident also in the index, incidentally (and most usefully) expanded some 50% to 78 3-column small-print pages. The reorganized table of contents has also been considerably expanded and improved. The actual articles were written by 200 authorities, 72 of them first time authors in this edition; many well-known, all with impressive academic credentials. A great many illustrations, diagrams including color plates, photomicrograhs and tables; up-to-date bibliographic references follow each article; there is a new system of cross-reference by chapter further facilitated by new running-head chapter numbers; in 22 parts with a total of 948 varying-length chapters including 5 new ones solely on treatment (antimicrobial; cytotoxic & immunosuppressant drugs; medical treatment of hormone-dependent cancer; respiratory failure management; and diet therapy in acute & hormone-chronic diseases). An exceptionally useful book not only for medical students and practitioners, but for all biomedical scientists.

REVIEW of T-2
from *TIC* (Oct. 1976), p. 6.

As Walsh McDermott puts it here: 'Medicine is not a science but a learned profession deeply rooted in a number of sciences and charged with the obligation to apply them for man's benefit'. This is true also of dentistry, which is a highly specialized branch of the art of medicine. With the emphasis today on the medical aspects of our profession, as opposed to the surgical, a classical text (it was first edited by Cecil and Loeb, a half century ago) such as this magnificent and complete textbook of medicine should be on every office shelf. Today's dentist increasingly looks to the problems of oral and systemic disease and turns to a new pharmacologic control of pain by psychosedation and other means. For all this the patient's medical history and health are essential and so a reference work—complete and up-to-date as this one—is needed. As Beeson himself writes in the section on The Nature of Medicine: 'I have not found it helpful (except as an editor!) to read a book like this in systematic cover-to-cover fashion . . . you should use it . . . as a place in which information can be obtained about problems being dealt with at the time'. It's all here, well written by experts. An essential!

REVIEW OF T-2
from *Annals of Internal Medicine* (1976), Vol. 84, pp. 109-110.
The Quadrennial rites are upon us again and a new edition, the 14th, of this well-known textbook of medicine is now available. The current preface pays respect to antecedent editors, indicates that there are 200 contributors to the present edition, of whom 72 are new, and states that a major goal is to give as much information as is practical about therapy. Five new chapters, solely about treatment have been added: 'Antimicrobial Therapy', 'Cytotoxic and Immunosuppressive Agents', 'Medical Treatment of Hormone-Dependent Cancers', 'Respiratory Failure and Its Management', and 'Diet Therapy in

Acute and Chronic Disease'. A new essay has also been added that deals with the care of the patient with terminal illness. All these are most appropriate and often needed by the many who turn to this book for advice. It is also appropriate for me to point out an error already noted by the authors and hopefully corrected in subsequent printings. This concerns the dosage of gentamycin and is in the sixth paragraph of the first column of page 315. This should now read 3 to 5 mg per kg body weight rather than 50 to 100 mg per kg body weight. Both the corrected dose of gentamycin and the dose of kanamycin in this paragraph apply to the 24 hour quantum. Furthermore the statements that concern digitalis on pages 820 (3rd paragraph) and 834 (6th paragraph) require further amplification, found in Chapter 541.

To whom is this book addressed? It now contains a staggering volume of information, so staggering that it is a reference textbook, for all practical purposes. The authors try to be all-encompassing, a state of affairs that we can well understand emotionally, but which must add little to the bread and butter clinical life led by most internists. It is not easy to wade through a miasma of information, seemingly written to emphasize the aridity of our so-called scientific language. The content is potentially exciting but the form tends to hide the exciting parts, rather like a shapeless shift draped over the Venus de Milo. I look back to the simple and beautiful writings of individuals like Ryle, as exemplified by his book on the natural history of disease. Somehow he gave life to the topic at hand and this cannot be said for many chapters of this book. Is there not some way of doing this or is it all so much window dressing? The sheer factual detail is awesome—note the classification of megoloblastic anemias—and the question arises as to how important it is to know 37 possible pathophysiologic approaches to hypoglycemia, most of which are so inordinately rare as to be seen once in a lifetime and then serendipitously recognized. It is agreed that we should know of their existence but analytically they are beyond most of us. It is of little import to state that the best mind is the prepared mind because it is virtually impossible to maintain a factually prepared mind these days. I often wonder whether such a textbook as this is one of the reasons for excessive investigation of a problem because 'all has not been excluded'.

This book obviously fulfills a most important function but a question that needs to be answered is whether it is to be considered a method of learning, a book of reference, or, by trying to be both, to fall between two stools. It may be that the time has come for large tomes such as this to diversify. There should be two editions. One would serve as a reference book, much as this particular one, and the other would be a condensation of the parent volume that includes only that information relevant to the more common diseases seen in the practice of occidental medicine. A major attempt should be made to make the condensation readable in the best sense of good literature.

In this instance no individual is capable of a review that can truly critically examine all the data presented, but a number of chapters were sampled by colleagues and the outcome was satisfactory. This book maintains the impeccable scientific content of its predecessors. I am delighted to have it by me; like an amulet it will give me a sense of security, like a sword of Damocles it will make me question that security, and like a spur it will goad me to further efforts in learning. (Thomas C. Gibson, M.B., M.R.C.P., University of Vermont College of Medicine, Burlington, Vermont)

REVIEW OF T-2
from *The Lancet* (Feb. 7, 1976), p. 285.

There must be daunting problems in producing new editions of this standard text, amongst them the trials of corresponding with 200 authors. In the latest edition, the first without Cecil and Loeb's names in the title, Dr. Beeson and Dr. McDermott solve most problems skilfully, and the book remains unequalled as a comprehensive reference work. The text has been thoroughly revised, and 72 contributors are new. Much more emphasis is given to practical matters of management, with five chapters devoted to difficult therapeutic areas. Those on antimicrobial drugs and on cytotoxic agents are especially useful additions. Balance is generally excellent, though sarcoidosis gets eleven pages while polyarteritis nodosa has only two. There are minor duplications (e.g., for obstructive cardiomyopathy and respiratory failure) and occasional peculiarities of organization; surely Sjogren's syndrome should be put with the connective-tissue disorders. The rising fortunes of immunology are reflected by a high place in the table of contents, but the title Immune Disease seems rather limiting for such a widely ranging subject. There are many other welcome additions—amongst them the sick-sinus syndrome, vascular disease of the intestine, primary immunodeficiency diseases, and neutrophil-dysfunction syndromes. The section of haematology and haemopoietic diseases is almost completely new, and Dr. R.L. Nachmann deserves great credit for this revision. Two of the finest, and wisest, chapters are those by the editors themselves— Beeson on becoming a clinician and McDermott on drugs and microbes. Future editions will need to take account of SI units. A chapter on drug interactions would be useful, as would more illustrations (e.g., drawings of congenital abnormalities). The word neurotic should be dropped from angio-oedema, and diseases based on immediate hypersensitivity deserve a section of their own. Some references cited in the text are not given in full. The format, cross-referencing, and index are all greatly improved.

REVIEW OF T-3
from *Delaware Medical Journal* (March 1978), Vol. 50, No. 3, p. 172.

The nineteenth edition of the textbook coming from Johns Hopkins is only about 200 pages longer than the eighteenth. The organization of the book is exactly the same as the eighteenth. Incidentally the table of contents is broken down into reasonable subject headings for anyone interested in using it as a starting point for a filing system of general medical information.

The book is very readable. The strength of the book is its charts and tables which present in summary form the information found in the narrative portion.

The book is a complete text for medicine although not encyclopedic; i.e. some of the most esoteric subjects are not mentioned, yet the general field of medicine is well covered. The purpose of republishing a text is, of course, to update the text in the light of medical advances. This has been well accomplished in this revision.

All in all this is an excellent text to provide the student with a good working knowledge of general internal medicine.

REVIEW OF T-3
from *Chest* (May 1977), Vol. 71, p. 28.

Principles and Practice of Medicine is a thorough and complete medical reference text. In particular, the opening chapters dealing with the approach to the patient and the discussion of the problems of collection and analysis of clinical information, conversing with patients and obtaining a history, the use of a clinical laboratory, and the approach to diagnoses are of general use to the medical student beginning his clinical experience.

Although the entire spectrum of medicine is covered in a comprehensive and thorough manner with up-to-date and pertinent information, there tends to be a variation in the overall quality and depth of analysis throughout the book. No doubt this is due to the large number of contributing authors and editors. Since it is difficult to critically assess a volume of this length, for me the most meaningful comment on the overall value of the book is that in comparing it to Harrison's *Textbook of Medicine* as a general medical reference, I found that on a number of occasions, after first consulting the *Principles and Practice of Medicine,* it was necessary to look to another medical reference source for additional information. Often, information not available in the book edited by Harvey et al. was concisely outlined in Harrison's *Text-*

book of Medicine, and, therefore, I personally would prefer Harrison's *Text-book of Medicine* as a general medical guide.

Steven R. Goldring, M.D.
Boston

REVIEW OF T-3
from *Annals of Internal Medicine* (1976), Vol. 85, pp. 699-700.

One might think that the 19th edition of a text, particularly one that follows the 18th by just 4 years, would be a comparatively simple update encompassing the advances within the interval. Some areas do little more than polish and amplify (Sections 6, 7, and 9), whereas others ('Psychiatry in Medicine'), have been completely rewritten. To some degree this reflects shifts in authorship among Johns Hopkins' faculty in keeping with the basic philosophy of this textbook to encompass the current medical practice of that one institution. Nevertheless, substantial change and addition have occurred as indicated by the fact that this edition has 242 pages, nine chapters, an appendix of normal laboratory values, and innumerable tables longer than its predecessor.

Unlike two other standard U.S. texts of medicine, *The Principles and Practice of Medicine* is not an encyclopedic display of the breadth of this field. At its best this text provides the physician a 'how to do it' approach to *diagnose and treat sick patients* rather than a compilation of diseases considered in isolation from physician or patient. Several of the new chapters are clearly included to facilitate further this approach: Chapter 1, 'The Collection and Analysis of Clinical Information'; and Chapter 22, 'Laboratory Evaluation of the Cardiovascular System'. Its theme is supported by having each section stress methods to acquire and interpret information as it may pertain to the whole patient, fluid and electrolyte balance, or a specific organ system. The best sections do not emphasize the acquisition of a global data base but rather the logical step-by-step development of knowledge through deductive process. In this regard, I particularly enjoyed the sections on diseases of the gastrointestinal tract, since the title and emphasis of each chapter therein relate to common chief complaints. Although this section was the one least changed from the previous edition, new summary tables and the newer diagnostic methods have been included. Surprisingly, those chapters emphasizing detailed pathophysiologic considerations of organ function seem rather out of character with the principal thrust of the book, since they appear to include more than what serves accurate diagnosis and therapy.

Some chapters just miss the mark, and deficiencies in the previous edition have not always been improved. The hematology section, to my view, had a unique opportunity to demonstrate an orderly, neat approach to the diagnosis and management of the anemias, but it bogs down by trying to catalog many varieties of disease; the section on nonmalignant white cell disorders is too sparse to have much impact.

Overall, this book is a remarkable achievement. To my knowledge, no other general textbook attempts to relate to the practice of medicine—as such, it presents practical clues on how to interpret laboratory values, X rays, or key symptoms; how to deal with drug dependence or sexual disorders; and how to diagnose and treat cardiopulmonary arrest or shock—and yet also provides classically authoritative sections such as that on medical genetics.

Perhaps I can best summarize by saying that this is a textbook of medicine that should be read from cover to cover and used thereafter whenever it becomes difficult to develop a cohesive diagnostic plan. It lacks depth in some areas, however, and the more encyclopedic general and specialty texts will be required to provide more detailed information.

John S. Thompson, M.D.
University of Iowa
Iowa City, Iowa

REVIEWS OF T-1, T-2, T-3
from *Medical Textbook Review,* Medical Sickness Annuity and Life Assurance Society Ltd., London, pp. 31-32.

T-1

This is the best of the large medical tomes. It is up-to-date, lively, lucid and nicely presented. Possibly too heavy for casual reading but in all excellent and ought to be considered by every medical student.

T-2

This is a recent edition of Cecil and Loeb's *Textbook of Medicine* first published in 1927. It is very thorough and covers all aspects of medicine including therapy. Over 200 authors have contributed to the present edition and although it is easy to use for reference it is not for bedtime reading. Good library material.

T-3

A mammoth American textbook of internal medicine representing the 'Johns Hopkins tradition' and having its origins in a work by Osler first published in 1892. This is a readable, up-to-date and fully comprehensive book containing a vast amount of information. The feature which makes it a winner is the inclusion of numerous summary tables scattered throughout the book. These alone will prove invaluable for medical students revising for Final M.B. and for M.R.C.P. candidates. A nice one and stupendous value at the price. There is also a separate self-assessment guide by Margoles, Harvey, Johns, Owens, and Ross.

REVIEWS OF T-1, T-2, T-3
from *Continuing Education for the Family Physician* (July 1978), p. 66

With the exception of its editors, a textbook of medicine is unlikely to be read cover-to-cover. Nevertheless, when the textbook's table of contents is well constructed, a reader may be attracted to browse in sections of the book. The tables of contents of the three books under consideration are likely to bring a reader into the book.

The books' origins and departures

Textbook of Medicine originated as Cecil's classic book (1927). The derivation of *Harrison's Principles of Internal Medicine,* as the title shows, began with Tinsley R. Harrison (1950), and *The Principles and Practice of Medicine* is a Hopkins-based outgrowth of the illustrious Sir William Osler's original work (1892).

Medical textbooks initially took an encyclopedic form from which they have moved to a larger perspective that is evident in their tables of contents. In other words, the books have become more patient-oriented as distinguished from disease-oriented. This fact is borne out in all three books under review, perhaps most strongly in *The Principles and Practice of Medicine.* At the same time, the books' value as a general reference source has been maintained.

The editors, contributing authors, and publishers of all three books have given the medical profession true masterpieces in the mixed art of writing, editing, and publishing. The books abound in superb illustrations and helpful tables. Typography and format enhance readability, a feature of no small importance to busy students and physicians. I cannot name one book as superior; I am delighted to have had access to all.

REVIEW OF P-3
from *Kirkus Reviews,* Vol. 39, July 1971.

Aside from the obvious (and it's hard to escape the obvious with Dr. Miller) remarks about checkups and preventive techniques, sound diet, exercise, the proper sleep and relaxation, the right working conditions, this incorporates a great deal of his stalwart *Complete Medical Guide* in a massive volume. It's hard to think of what might have been overlooked: the body, with all its organs and senses; mental health; marriage and your sex life; having children and bringing them up; and at the end there are many 'disease scenarios' ranging from purpura to suicide or motion sickness. You can't get in trouble with Dr. Miller (he takes a firm stand on smoking, drugs, etc.) but then he can rarely get in trouble either since he's descriptive rather than prescriptive and sidesteps controversies such as the pill. He also is careful to refer you to your own doctor, and if you have a family doctor at hand, you should have better than the equivalent of Dr. Miller.

REVIEW OF P-3
from *Science Books,* American Association for the Advancement of Science, Vol. 8, No. 1, May 1972.

This is the first printing of a book intended for family use as an aid to healthful living. There are six parts to the book. Part one concerns the nature of preventive medicine. Part two deals with preventive therapy, such as weight control, sleep, and drugs. Part three mentions care of one's body including the skin, hair, and nails and various systems such as circulatory system and endocrine glands. Part four is involved with mental health and refers to help for mental and emotional problems and preventive psychiatry. Part five on preventive family care concerns such items as healthy adjustment in marriage and preventive medicine for children. Part six, disease scenarios, lists 63 diseases from Addison's disease and aging to ulcerative colitis and varicose veins. The three outstanding chapters are those concerned with preventive body care, mental health, and the family, respectively. Part five on preventive family care is especially instructive for young adults concerned with marriage and raising a family. The chapter on disease scenarios is acceptable for general reference purposes. This book is best for collateral reading and reference.

REVIEW OF P-3
from *Library Journal,* Vol. 96, No. 13, July 1971.

'Treatment never equals prevention. . . . It is prevention that must be counted upon to make the big inroads against death and disability'. Thus the theme of this volume on preventive medicine for the home, which emphasizes health rather than just absence of disease. It covers general health care, care of the body systems, and preventive mental care. The section on family preventive care includes chapters on sexual adjustment and genetic counseling. Over 60 'disease scenarios' conclude the volume. Each scenario emphasizes the dynamic nature of the physician's diagnosis and treatment, and includes the epidemiology, treatment, and prognosis of the disease, as well as up-to-date advice on prevention. Helpful and frequent cross references enhance the text. The broad coverage, the positive emphasis, and the nontechnical vocabulary make this a volume to be recommended highly. Shirley B. Heaalein, State University of New York Library, Buffalo.

REVIEW OF P-3
from *Choice,* Association of College and Research Libraries, American Library Association, Vol. 8, No. 10, Dec. 1971.

Appeals to a nurse-teacher of student nurses because curriculum focus should be prevention of disease and teaching good health to our community—something this book does for the public. The authors are well qualified, as is apparent from their treatment of health and the disease scenarios. The public will appreciate the use of medical terminology followed by definitions which they often hear from their own doctors—minus the definitions. The short paragraphs with topic headings make for easy reading. Will appeal especially to parents with young families and give excellent background to readers with no formal biological training which so many people lack, yet need, today. It is a matter-of-fact presentation which psychologically helps many people to accept themselves. The bibliographic references in the mental health section are a good feature. All in all, a good book for any family.

REVIEW OF P-4
from *Stanley News and Press,* Albermarle, N.C., July 27, 1976.

This is the health book you've been waiting for.
    From sniffles to terminal cancer, it deals with the common health ailments

mankind is subject to contract—symptoms and causes, treatment and cure, and, best of all, proven methods for preventing these diseases and ailments from occurring. Throughout, the guideline emphasis is on prevention, then on the best way to handle illness if it should strike.

This 6 by 9 book is 2½ inches thick and weighs over 3 pounds. It contain 277 chapters in 63 major sections. Listing of the contents requires 10 pages; the index, 20 pages.

More than 75 percent of the material in TEOCD is new, updated from the original edition to meet the latest authoritative disclosures in the rapidly changing field of medicine.

Quoting from the introduction:

'Every person is responsible for his own health. He must learn how his body works and what can threaten its functioning. The person who identifies these threats and tries to avoid them is taking the most important steps there are in battling disease. This book outlines these steps in a useful, understandable manner . . . as a rule, health comes from the way people live, not from doctors and hospitals. This book is a blueprint for better, more healthful living'.

Also, the introduction forthrightly warns: 'In the face of serious illness, no book, however thorough it might be, can take the place of consultation with a physician'.

This is certainly one of the best, if not the best, useful and practical health books you can find—one that every individual and every family can use to great benefit.

Fred T. Morgan

REVIEW OF P-4
from *Choice*, Dec. 1976.

A unique feature of this comprehensive handbook is that it stresses the prevention of various diseases and physical conditions by providing guidelines for better health through improved habits of living. The range of diseases and physical conditions covered is great, and the handbook should be a very valuable addition to the libraries of modern families. Undoubtedly it will be sought by many family members as a reference source in their community libraries. Among the topics included are alcoholism, arthritis, childhood diseases, the ears and hearing, flu, headache, mononucleosis, teeth and gums, and weight problems. This voluminous work is not intended to serve as a medical book nor as a 'doctor-book' but rather as an educational tool for readers who are interested in an increased understanding of their own bodies and the relationships between health and disease. The editors point out that no book can replace professional medical consultation. Rather, the book provides knowledge that can assist in the development of an enlightened, responsible doctor-patient relationship. New knowledge supplants the earlier edition of the encyclopedia, and this work largely covers new material. An underlying assumption of the editors is that the use of natural modes of disease prevention, such as diet and exercise, are best. From the point of view of a family social scientist, the book is a practical and easy-to-read guide for families who are interested in an important aspect of family life and good health.

REVIEW OF P-4
from Baltimore, Md. *Morning Sun,* Oct. 31, 1977.

This 1,296-page hardcover is like an old-fashioned family doctor; it talks about many common ailments and tells how some natural remedies may provide a cure or preventative. It emphasizes the role of diet and exercise, often ignored by doctors addicted to prescription drugs.

REVIEW OF P-4
from *American Reference Book Annual,* 1977.

Beginning with alcoholism and ending with weight problems, the 63 sections in this volume cover the major diseases and disorders that afflict men, women, and children. The 63 sections are composed of 277 chapters. There are as few as one chapter per section (e.g. appendix, bronchitis, celiac disease) as well as sections that contain many chapters (e.g. allergy has six chapters, arthritis has eleven, insomnia has nine). The underlying philosophy of this encyclopedic work is 'natural is best'. The easy-to-read nontechnical approach should appeal to the layperson. The editors have done a good job of explaining how to prevent disease and the best way to handle illness if it should occur. Causes and symptoms of hundreds of health problems from autism to zinc deficiency are fully explained, with recent information on treatment and/or cure, and with emphasis on prevention. The sections on cancer, heart disease, and emotional and nervous disorders are quite extensive and well written, and they include recent references from medical and scientific monographs and journals. The index is extensive and includes cross references. This volume can and should be read by most individuals, who will be better informed patients when they next visit their physicians.

James E. Bobick

REVIEW OF P-4
from *San Francisco Review of Books,* San Francisco, Calif., Nov. 1976.

Among the gigantic volumes on gardening and health offered us by the Rodale Press is *The Encyclopedia of Common Diseases.* The editors believed that health 'comes from the way people live, not from doctors and hospitals'. To show that the editors are not without a sense of humor, they offer this advice on the subject of elimination: '. . . try to relax. Pick up a magazine or a book . . . Stay for about ten minutes . . . it has been said that toilet bowls themselves can cause problems by being too high. . . . feet should be firmly planted upon the ground (floor) to induce a proper bowel movement . . . put a stack of old books under each foot, or keep a footstool (pun unintentional) nearby'.

The Editors

REVIEW OF P-4
from *Independent Press,* Jan. 26, 1977.

A major argument against so many of the books on health and diet is that the authors lead the reader to believe that whatever disease they may be suffering from—diabetes, cancer, or colitis, has a single cause, frequently the lack of a particular vitamin or trace mineral. The ENCYCLOPEDIA sometimes tends in this direction, such as its lengthy discussion of the deficiency of chromium as a major cause of diabetes, but the book makes no specific claims in its examination of the evidence for a number of possible causes, enlarging on the factors of most importance.

It's a helpful source for sorting out the claims of various books and articles on health, diet, and food supplements and for giving the reader guidance on maintaining health, particularly through proper diet.

D.H. Stefanson

REVIEW OF P-4
from *Jackson, Tenn. Sun,* July 11, 1976.

For more than a quarter of a century, Prevention magazine has emphasized the necessity of not only treating diseases correctly, but also treating one's body properly to keep the disease from occurring in the first place.

Carrying this theme through in a text arranged alphabetically by names of the body afflicted and names of the diseases that bother us all, the editors have developed an excellent daily reference work that is written in layman's language.

The advice is direct, for example on anemia: 'By all means include iron-rich foods in your diet . . . this is nature's way, and no one has yet come up with anything better'. Then follows a list of foods high in iron.

The advice is thorough too. In the section on arthritis, the writers discuss every form of therapy from vitamin C to X-rays to raw foods to ultraviolet rays to cherry juice to personality quirks. . . . Each section is authoritative, not speculative, and research findings are summarized with a minimum of scholarly language.

Got sinus problems? Alcoholic consumption and smoking are two of your worst enemies, because they destroy the body's natural abilities to combat this persistent nuisance.

Danny Walker

REVIEW OF P-4
from *Garden City, N.Y. Newsday,* June 20, 1977.

The Encyclopedia of Common Diseases (Rodale Press, $20), by the staff of Prevention Magazine, is billed as a comprehensive handbook of disease symptoms, treatment and prognosis, written for the layman. It also includes information on prevention of diseases, as well as some natural remedies not often prescribed by traditional practitioners, and in-depth chapters on such topics as heart disease, cancer, arthritis, and emotional disorders.

REVIEW OF P-4
from *Independent Review Service,* Baltimore, Md. 21236, Dec. 14, 1976.

THE ENCYCLOPEDIA OF COMMON DISEASES by the staff of Prevention magazine. . . .an incredible book, almost 1,300 pages in length. Covers a wide array of illnesses, their causes, and offers practical organic solutions in most cases. Indexed. (Roadale: $19.95)

Rickey Shanklin

REVIW OF P-4
from *Daily Record*, Morris County, N.J., Aug. 8, 1976.

'The Encyclopedia of Common Diseases' *($19.95, Rodale Press, Inc.)* by the staff of Prevention Magazine sounds like it belongs in a physician's office, but it belongs in the home of every family and every person concerned with the maintenance of good health. I have seen no finer, comparable book of its kind in years. It is a total guide to preventing, recognizing, and dealing with all forms of health problems.

Alan Caruba

REVIEW OF P-4
from *San Francisco, Calif. Chronicle*, July 26, 1976.

ASK THE DOCTOR

MEDICAL BOOKS FOR THE HOME
By Robert Mendelsohn, M.D.

DEAR DR. MENDELSOHN: What medical books should be on my book-shelf?
D.M.

Get hold of a standard medical textbook that emphasizes disease management, such as the latest edition of 'Current Therapy' edited by the distinguished Howard F. Conn, M.D. (W.B. Saunders, $21). You should also have one of the anti-establishment books, an excellent example of which is the 'Encyclopedia of Common Diseases' by the staff of Prevention Magazine (Rodale Press, $19.95).

Do your best to obtain a Physician's Desk Reference (available only from Medical Economics, Box. 58, Oradell, N.J. 07649, $15).

An excellent source book for drug interaction is 'Hazards of Medication' by Eric W. Martin (J.B. Lippincott, $32). Three books that take a critical look at modern medical care are 'The Medicine Men' by Leonard Tushnet, M.D. (St. Martin's Press, $7.95), 'Medical Nemesis' by Ivan Illich (Pantheon, $8.95) and 'Presymptomatic Detection and Early Diagnosis: A Critical Appraisal' by C.L. Sharp and Harry Kenn (Williams and Wilkins, $19.95).

REVIEW OF P-5

from *American Reference Book Annual 1975,* ed. by Bohdan S. Wymar. Littleton, Co.: Libraries Unlimited Inc., 1975.

This book is divided into two distinct parts. The first consists of 34 chapters, each on a special phase of medical care. The second part is an encyclopedia that briefly defines and describes medical terms and diseases. The author, a well-known physician, editor, and writer, has written over 40 books, some of them bestselling medical guides. This title is well written and authentic, but it is unfortunately a bit too brief and elementary for many readers. It is probably worth the small price, however, and may be of value in the home library if the price of a more comprehensive publication is prohibitive. One of the author's other guides, such as the *Modern Home Medical Adviser* (Doubleday, 1969), is preferable for many readers. Better still is the *Stein and Day International Medical Encyclopedia* (Stein and Day, 1971).

Theodora Andrews

Biographical Data on Editors or Authors of Books of Medical Instruction

a. TEXTBOOKS OF MEDICINE

1. *Biography of George Widmer Thorn,*[1] *Editor of T-1*

Born:
January 15, 1906 in Buffalo, New York

Education:
M.D., University of Buffalo, 1929

Honorary degrees:
A.M. Harvard, 1942
D.Sc., Temple University, 1951
D.Sc., Suffolk University, 1961
D.Sc., College of Wooster, 1964
D.Sc., New York Medical College, 1972
LL.D., Dalhousie University, 1950
LL.D., Queen's University, 1954
D. Med., Catholic University Louvain, 1960
M.D., Geneva

Professional experience:
House Officer, Millard Fillmore Hospital, Buffalo, New York, 1929-1930
Assistant, Department of Physiology, University of Buffalo, 1931-1932
Instructor, Department of Medicine, University of Buffalo, 1932-1934
Rockefeller Fellow in Medicine, Harvard Medical School and Massachusetts
    General Hospital, Boston, 1934-1935
Assistant Professor of Physiology, Ohio State University, 1935-1936
Rockefeller Fellow in Medicine, Johns Hopkins Medical School, 1936-1937
Associate in Medicine, Johns Hopkins Medical School, 1937-1938
Read Ellsworth Fellow in Medicine, Johns Hopkins Medical School, 1938

Associate Professor of Medicine, Johns Hopkins Medical School, 1938-1942
Assistant Physician, Johns Hopkins Hospital, 1937-1939
Associate Physician, Johns Hopkins Hospital, 1939-1942
Hersey Professor of Theory and Practice of Physic, Harvard Medical School, 1942-1972
Emeritus Professor, Harvard Medical School, 1972-
Samuel A. Levine Professor of Medicine, 1967-1972
Samuel A. Levine Emeritus Professor, 1972-
Physician-in-Chief, Peter Bent Brigham Hospital, 1942-1972; now Emeritus
Hugh J. Morgan Visiting Professor, Vanderbilt University, 1967
Visiting Professor of Medicine, Columbia College of Physicians and Surgeons, 1968
Visiting Professor of Medicine, Cornell Medical School and New York Hospital, 1970
Wingate Johnson Visiting Professor, Bownman Gray School of Medicine, Wake Forest University, 1972
Consulting Internist, Boston Psychopathic Hospital, 1943-
Member of Research and Development Advisory Board, Smith, Kline and French Laboratories, 1953-1969
Consultant, Children's Medical Center, U.S.P.H.S., and U.S. Army Medical Services Graduate School
Member, Committee on Stress, National Research Council
Member, National Advisory Committee on Radiation, 1958-
Member, Drug Research Board, National Research Council and National Academy of Sciences, 1972
Member of the Corporation, Massachusetts Institute of Technology
Editor-in-Chief, Medcom Faculty of Medicine, 1972-

Awards:
Chancellor's Medal, University of Buffalo, 1943.
Osler Oration Award, Canadian Medical Association, 1949
U.S. Pharmaceutical Manufacturers' Association Award, 1951
Alverenga Award, 1951
John Phillips Memorial Award, American College of Physicians, 1955
Dr. Charles V. Chapin Memorial Award, American Medical Association, 1956
George Miniot Award, American Medical Association, 1963
Oscar B. Hunter Memorial Award, American Therapeutic Society, 1967

Memberships:
Diplomate, American Board of Internal Medicine
Fellow, Royal College of Physicians (London, England)

Fellow, American College of Physicians
American Society for Clinical Investigation (Emeritus)
American Medical Association (Gold Medallist, 1932, 1939)
Association of American Physicians (President, 1970)
American Physiological Society
Endocrine Society (President, 1962)
American Clinical and Climatological Association (President)
American Academy of Arts and Sciences
Royal Society of Medicine (Honorary)
Interurban Clinical Club
Johns Hopkins Society of Scholars

2. *Biography of Paul Bruce Beeson,*[2] *Coeditor of T-2*

Born:
October 18, 1908 in Livingston, Montana

Education:
University of Washington, 1925-1928
M.D., C.M., McGill University, 1933

Honorary degrees:
D.Sc., Emory University, 1968
D.Sc., McGill University, 1971
D.Sc., Albany Medical College, 1975
D.Sc., Yale University, 1975

Professional experience:
Assistant, Rockefeller Institute, 1937-1939
Assitant, Harvard Medical School, 1939-1940
Assistant Professor of Medicine, Emory University Medical School, 1942-
    1946; Professor, Chairman of the Department, 1946-1952
Ensign Professor of Medicine, Chairman of the Department of Internal
    Medicine, Yale Medical School, 1952-1965
Physician-in-Chief, University Service, Grace-New Haven Community Hospital,
    1952-1965
Visiting Investigator, Wright-Fleming Institute of Microbiology, London,
    1958-1959
Nuffield Professor of Clinical Medicine, Oxford University, 1965-1974
Professor of Medicine, University of Washington, Seattle, 1974-
Distinguished Physician, Veterans' Administration, 1974-

Memberships:
National Academy of Science
American Academy of Arts and Science
American College of Physicians
Society of Experimental Biology and Medicine
American Society for Clinical Investigation
Association of American Physicians (President 1967)
Association of Physicians of Great Britain and Ireland

Research:
Infectious Diseases
Immunology
Clinical Medicine

3.   *Biography of Walsh McDermott,*[3] *Coeditor of T-2*

Born:
October 24, 1909 in New Haven, Connecticut

Education:
B.A., Princeton University, 1930
M.D., Columbia University, 1934

Honorary degrees:
D.Sc., Princeton University, 1974
D.Sc., Dartmouth College, 1976

Professional experience:
Intern; Assistant Resident, New York Hospital, 1934-1937
Instructor; Associate Professor of Medicine, New York Hospital, 1937-1955
Livingston Farrand Professor; Chairman of the Department of Public Health,
   Cornell University Medical College, 1955-1972
Professor of Public Affairs in Medicine, Cornell University Medical College,
   1972-1975
Emeritus Professor of Public Affairs in Medicine, Cornell University Medical
   College, 1975-
Trustee, Columbia University, 1973-
Special Advisor to Robert Wood Johnson Foundation, 1972-

Awards and honors:
Lasker Award, American Public Health Association, 1955
Dyer Award, 1959
National Institute of Health First International Lectureship Award, 1963
Trudeau Medal, 1963
Woodrow Wilson Award, Princeton University, 1969

Memberships:
National Academy of Science
American Academy of Arts and Science
National Institute of Medicine
American Society of Clinical Investigation
Association of American Physicians
Council on Foreign Relations
Interurban Clinical Club
Honorable Fellow of the Royal College of Physicians

Research:
Public Health

4. *Biography of Abner McGehee Harvey,*[4] *Editor of T-3*

Born:
July 30, 1911 in Little Rock, Arkansas

Education:
A.B., Washington and Lees University, 1930
M.D., Johns Hopkins University, 1934

Honorary degrees:
D.Sc., Washington and Lee University, 1949
D.Sc., University of Arkansas, 1951
D.Sc., Medical College of Ohio, 1976

Professional experience:
Intern, Johns Hopkins Hospital, 1934-1935
Assistant Resident, Johns Hopkins Hospital, 1935-1937
Research Fellow, National Institute of Medical Research, London, 1937-1939
Fellow, Johnson Foundation for Biophysics, University of Pennsylvania, 1939-1940

Resident Physician, Johns Hopkins Hospital, 1940-1941
Professor of Medicine, Johns Hopkins Medical School; Physician-in-Chief,
   Johns Hopkins Hospital, 1946-1973

Awards:
R.H. Williams Award, 1975

Memberships:
Fellow of the American Academy of Arts and Sciences
American Rheumatism Association
Association of American Physicians (President, 1968)
American Society for Clinical Investigation (President, 1956)
Physiological Society of Great Britain
Interurban Clinical Club
American Physiological Soceity
American Clinical and Climatological Association (President, 1971)
American College of Physicians
American Society for Pharmaceutical and Experimental Therapeutics
Association of Professors of Medicine (President, 1960)
American Osler Society (President, 1976)

Research:
Neurophysiology
Clinical Therapeutics

b.   POPULAR HOME MEDICAL BOOKS

1.   *Biography of Morris Fishbein,*[5] *Editor of P-5*

Born:
July 22, 1889 in St. Louis, Missouri

Education:
B.S., University of Chicago, 1910
M.D., Rush Medical College, 1912

Honorary degrees:
D. Pharmacy, Rutgers University, 1942
LL.D., Florida South College, 1957
D.Sc., Chicago Medical School, 1965

Professional experience:
Fellow in Pathology, Rush Medical College, 1912
Assistant editor to editor, *Journal of the American Medical Association,* 1913-1949
Editor of *Hygeia,* until 1949
Editor of *Bulletin of Society of Medical History,* Chicago
Contributing editor, *Postgraduate Medicine,* 1950-1970
Member-in-chief of board of editors of *Exerpta Medica,* 1949-1971
Editor of *Medical World News,* 1960-1975
Medical Editor of *Family Health Magazine,* 1969-
Chairman of science advisory board, Municipal Tuberculosis Sanatorium and City of Hope
Professor Emeritus of Medicine, University of Illinois College of Medicine
Editor of medical section, *Britannica Book of the Year,* 1938-1972
Contributing editor of *McCall's Magazine,* 1959-1967

Awards:
Decorated Knight Commander Order of Crown of Italy
National Order of Merit of Carlos J. Finlay (Cuba)
Certificate of Merit from President Truman, 1948
Commander of the Civil Order of Health (Spain), 1952
Officer's Cross Order Orange-Nassau, Netherlands, 1954
Commander Cross of the Royal Order of Phoenix (Greece), 1967
Recipient of the Jesse L. Rosenberger medal for achievements in public medicine and medical education, University of Chicago, 1968
Willard Thompson medal, American Gerontology Society, 1972

Memberships:
Member of several professional advertising committees and organizations
Fellow of the American Public Health Association
Member of A.A.A.S., Phi Delta Epsilon, Alpha Omega Alpha, Sigma Delta Chi
Clubs: Variety, Lotus, Chicago Literary Club, Quardrangle, The Tavern, Standard, Arts

Author:
Numerous books, 1925-. Later ones include:
Joseph Bolivar DeLee, Crusading Obstetrician (with Sol Theron DeLee), 1949;
Handy Home Medical Adviser, 1972

Editor:
Numerous books and reports. Later ones include:

Modern Family Health Guide, 1967;
Heart Care, 1960;
Modern Home Medical Adviser, 1969;
Morris Fishbein, M.D., Autobiography, 1969

Died:
September 1976

NOTES

1. Source: *Who's Who in America,* 39th ed., 1976-1977. Vol. 2, Chicago, Marquis Who's Who, 1977, p. 3136.
2. Sources: *Who's Who in America,* 40th edition, 1978-1979. Vol. 1, p. 225; *Who's Who in Health Care,* 1st ed., New York: Hanover, 1977, p. 39.
3. Sources: *Who's Who in America,* 40th edition, 1978-1979, Chicago: Marquis Who's Who, Vol. 2, p. 2160; *Who's Who in Health Care,* 1st ed. New York: Hanover, 1977, p. 387.
4. Source: *Who's Who in America,* 40th edition, 1978-1979, Vol. 1, p. 1410.
5. Source: *Who's Who in America,* 39th edition, 1976-1977, Vol. 1, p. 1006.

Other Books in Print by Editors or Authors of Books of Medical Instruction

a. BY EDITORS OF TEXTBOOKS OF MEDICINE[1]

1. *Books by Editor of T-1*

Thorn, G.W.
  (editor) *Harrison's Principles of Internal Medicine*, 8th ed., New York: McGraw-Hill, 1977.

2. *Books by Editors of T-2*

Beeson, P.B. and W. McDermott,
  (editors) *Textbook of Medicine,* 14th ed., Philadelphia: Saunders, 1975.

3. *Books by Editor of T-3*

Harvey, A.M.
  Osler's Textbook Revisited. New York: Appleton-Century-Crofts, 1967.
  (with James Bordley) *Differential Diagnosis: The Interpretation of Clinical Evidence,* 2nd ed. Philadelphia: Saunders, 1970.
  Abridged ed., 1972.
  (with James Bordley) *Two Centuries of American Medicine.* Philadelphia: Saunders, 1976.
  (editor) *The Principles and Practice of Medicine,* 19th ed. New York: Appleton-Century-Crofts, 1976.
  Adventures in Medical Research: A Century of Discovery at Johns Hopkins. Baltimore: Johns Hopkins University Press, 1977.

b.   BY EDITORS OR AUTHORS OF POPULAR HOME MEDICAL BOOKS[3]

1.   *Books by Editor of P-1*

Cooley, Donald G.
  Science Book of Wonder Drugs. New York: Arno, 1954.
  *Better Homes and Gardens Family Medical Guide, rev. ed. Ed. by D.G.
  Cooley. New York: Meredith, 1977.

2.   *Books by Editor of P-2*

Homola, Samuel, D.C.
  Muscle Training for Athletes. Englewood Cliffs, N.J.: Prentice-Hall, 1968.
  Chiropractor's Treasury of Health Secrets. Englewood Cliffs, N.J.:
  Prentice-Hall, 1970.
  Secrets of Naturally Youthful Health and Vitality. Englewood Cliffs, N.J.:
  Prentice-Hall, 1971.
  *Doctor Homola's Natural Health Remedies. West Nyack, N.Y.: Parker,
  1973.
  Doctor Homola's Fat-Disintegrator Diet. Englewood Cliffs, N.J.: Prentice-
  Hall, 1977.
  (with Peter Lupas) *Peter Lupas' Guide to Radiant Health and Beauty:
  Mission Possible for Women.* Englewood Cliffs, N.J.: Prentice-Hall, 1977.

3.   *Books by Editors of P-3*

(i)   Miller, Benjamin F., M.D.
  When Doctors are Patients (Max Pinner, ed.). Philadelphia: R. West, 1952.
  (and Ruth Goode) *Man and His Body.* New York: Simon and Schuster,
  1960.
  Complete Medical Guide, rev. ed. New York: Simon and Schuster, 1967.
  (et al.) *Masculinity and Femininity.* New York: Houghton Mifflin, 1971.
  (and Lawrence Galton) **The Family Book of Preventive Medicine: How
  to Stay Well all the Time.* New York: Simon and Schuster, 1971.
  (et al.) *Freedom from Heart Attacks.* New York: Simon and Schuster,
  1972.
  (and Claire B. Keane) *Encyclopedia and Dictionary of Medicine and Nurs-
  ing.* Philadelphia: W.B. Saunders, 1972.

(and John T. Burt) *Good Health,* 3rd ed. Philadelphia: W.B. Saunders, 1972.

(et al.) *Investigating Your Health.* New York: Houghton Mifflin, 1974.

(ii) Galton, Lawrence

(with Benjamin F. Miller, M.D.) **The Family Book of Preventive Medicine: How to Stay Well all the Time.* New York: Simon and Schuster, 1971.

The Silent Disease: Hypertension. New York: Crown, 1973.

Don't Give Up on an Aging Parent. New York: Crown, 1975.

How Long Will I Live? And 434 Other Questions Your Doctor Doesn't Have Time to Answer and You Can't Afford to Ask. New York: Macmillan, 1976.

(with Broda Barnes) *Hypothyroidism: The Unsuspected Illness.* New York: Crowell, 1976.

Medical Advances: Over 300 Proven New Medical Treatments That May be of Help to You. New York: Crown, 1977.

Save Your Stomach. New York: Crown, 1977.

The Complete Book of Symptoms and What They Can Mean. New York: Simon and Schuster, 1978.

(with Oscar Roth) *Heart Attack: A Question and Answer Book.* New York: Lippincott, 1978.

Complete Medical Fitness and Health Guide for Men. New York: Simon and Schuster, 1979.

(with Laurence Friedman) *Freedom from Backaches.* New York: Pocketbooks, no date.

4. *Books by Editor of P-4*

Gerras, Charles

The Natural Way to Healthy Skin. Emmaus, Pennsylvania: Rodale, 1973.

(et al.) **The Encyclopedia of Common Diseases.* Emmaus, Pennsylvania: Rodale, 1976.

5. *Books by Editor of P-5*

Fishbein, Morris, M.D.

Popular Medical Encyclopedia. New York: Doubleday, 1946.

The New Illustrated Medical and Health Encyclopedia, unified ed., 18 vols. New York: Stuttman, 1970.

Medical Writing: The Technic and the Art, 4th ed. Springfield, Ill.: C.C. Thomas, 1972.

The Medical Follies. New York: AMS Press, 1976. Reprint of 1925 ed.

Fads and Quackery in Healing. New York: AMS Press, 1976. Rpt. of 1932 ed.

Modern Home Dictionary of Medical Words. New York: Doubleday, 1976.

The New Medical Follies. New York: AMS Press, 1977. Rpt. of 1927 ed.

(editor) *The New Illustrated Medical and Health Encyclopedia.* Family Health Guide Edition. New York: Stuttman, 1966.

The New Illustrated Medical and Health Encyclopedia. Spanish Language Edition. 2 vols. New York: Stuttman, 1967.

Modern Home Medical Adviser: Your Health and How to Preserve It. New York: Doubleday, 1969.

*The Handy Home Medical Adviser and Concise Medical Encyclopedia, new rev. ed. New York: Doubleday, 1973.

The New Illustrated Medical and Health Encyclopedia, 4 vols. Milwaukee: Purnell, 1975.

(and Justine Fishbein) *Fishbein's Illustrated Medical and Health Encyclopedia,* 4 vols. New York: Stuttman, 1977.

Doctors at War. New York: Arno. Rpt of 1945 ed. (s.d.).

History of the American Medical Association, 1847-1947. Rpt. of 1947 ed. Milwood, New York: Kraus Reprint Co. (s.d.).

Subsequent to compiling the above data, the writer discovered a more comprehensive source of listings of published works by the authors or editors of the books selected for this investigation. This source is the Library of Congress *National Union Catalogue* (pre-1956 imprints and subsequent volumes up to September, 1979). According to this source, the numbers of published works authored, edited, coauthored or coedited by the authors or editors of the selected books (excluding articles, translations or new editions of previous works), are as follows (see Table 60):

Table 60. *Numbers of books published by authors or editors of selected books of medical instruction*

Editor or author	Selected book	Tot. no. published books
G.W. Thorn, M.D.	T-1	3
P.B. Beeson, M.D.	T-2	2
W. McDermott, M.D.	T-2	3
A.M. Harvey, M.D.	T-3	5

contd.

Table 60 (*contd.*)

Editor or author	Selected book	Tot. no. published books
D.G. Cooley	P-1	16
S. Homola, D.C.	P-2	9
B. Miller, M.D.	P-3	14
L. Galton	P-3	19
C. Gerras	P-4	7
M. Fishbein, M.D.	P-5	79

Textbook average = (approximately) 3 books per editor
Popular average   = (approximately) 22 books per author or editor

NOTES

1. As appearing in *Medical Books and Serials in Print 1979: An Index to Literature in the Health Sciences,* New York: Bowker, 1979.
2. Titles of books investigated in the present study have been indicated by an asterisk.
3. As appearing in *Medical Books and Serials in Print 1979.*

Graph 60.   *Numbers of books published by authors or editors of selected books of medical instruction*

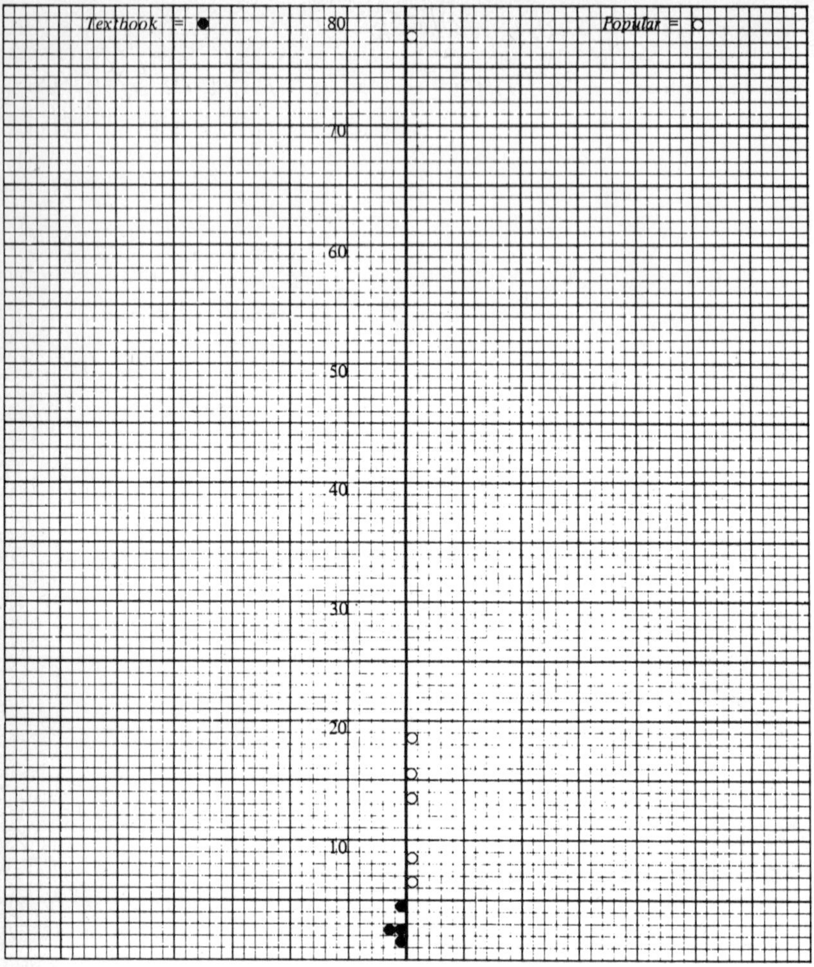

Osler's *The Principles and Practice of Medicine:* Some Historical Perspectives

a. SCHEMA OF DISEASE DESCRIPTION OF DIABETES MELLITUS[1]
(from Osler's *The Principles and Practice of Medicine,* 7th edition, 1909)

Definition

Etiology
  Incidence
  Hereditary Influences
  Sex
  Race
  Obesity
  Nervous Influences
  Injury
  Experimental Diabetes

Metabolism in Diabetes

Morbid Anatomy

The Pancreas in Diabetes

Symptoms
  The Urine
  Blood in Diabetes
  Diabetes in Children

Complications
  Cutaneous
  Pulmonary
  Renal
  Nervous System

Course

Diagnosis

Prognosis

Treatment
  Diet
  Medicinal Treatment

b. TABLES OF CONTENTS
(Major Headings) of Osler's *The Principles and Practice of Medicine* (1) 1st edition, 1892 and (2) 7th edition, 1909.[2]

1. *1st edition, 1892*

Specific infectious diseases
Constitutional diseases
Diseases of the digestive system
Diseases of the respiratory system
Diseases of the circulatory system
Diseases of the blood and ductless glands
Diseases of the nervous system
Diseases of the muscles
The intoxications: sun-stroke; obesity
Diseases due to animal parasites

2. *7th edition, 1909*

Diseases due to animal parasites
Specific infectious diseases
The intoxications and sun-stroke
Constitutional diseases
Diseases of the digestive system
Diseases of the respiratory system
Diseases of the kidneys
Diseases of the blood and ductless glands
Diseases of the circulatory system
Diseases of the nervous system
Diseases of the muscles

NOTES

1. Abner McGehee Harvey and Victor A. McKusick, *Osler's Textbook Revisited*, (New York: Appleton, 1967), pp. 179-195; also see pp. 196-197 for an evaluation of Osler's description of diabetes in light of current knowledge about the disease.
2. Harvey and McKusick 1967: 10.

Key Headings in Two Books Devoted to the Topic of Diabetes Mellitus

a. 'TEXTBOOK' TYPE: *JOSLIN'S DIABETES MELLITUS*

The following 'key headings' include all 32 chapter headings (see Arabic numerals) and all bold-type headings dispersed throughout the chapters (indicated by alphabetical letters).

1. CURRENT CONCEPTS OF DIABETES
    a. *Definition*
    b. *Classification of Diabetes*
    c. *The Origins of Diabetes*
        Hereditary Aspects
        Basic Defect and the Evolution of Diabetes
    d. *Stages of the Diabetic State*
        Chemical Diabetes
        Overt Diabetes
    e. *Dynamic Character of the Diabetic State*
    f. *Vascular Abnormalities in Prediabetes*
    g. *Relation Between the Metabolic Defect and Vascular Disease*
        Basic Considerations
        Clinical Application

2. EPIDEMIOLOGY AND DETECTION OF DIABETES
    a. *Epidemiology*
        — Frequency
            Primary Characteristics of the Data
        — Prevalence
            Prevalence of Diabetes in the United States
            Estimated Prevalence Outside the United States
        — Incidence of Diabetes
        — Influences on the Onset of Diabetes
            Statistical Genetics

Biochemical Genetics
Obesity
Trauma
Emotional Factors
b. *Detection of Diabetes*
   — Diabetic Detection Problems
   — Detection Screening—Technical Considerations
   — Screening Test Pitfalls and Problems
   — Results of Diabetes Detection Programs
      Very Select Population Studies
      Diabetes Detection with State, County, and Community
      Programs
      Diabetes Detection in Foreign Countries

3. PATHOPHYSIOLOGY OF DIABETES MELLITUS
a. *Diabetic Syndromes*
      The Acute Diabetic Syndrome
      The Chronic Diabetic Syndrome
      Regional Variants of the Diabetic Syndrome
      Lipoatrophic Diabetes
      Genetic Homogeneity or Heterogeneity of Diabetic Syn-
      dromes
b. *Endocrine Defects in Diabetes Mellitus*
      Diabetes in Man
c. *Insulin*
   — Chemistry
   — Antigenicity of Insulin
   — Immunologically Induced Experimental Insulitis
   — Biosynthesis
   — Storage
   — Glucose Metabolism of Islet Tissue
   — Insulin Secretion and Release
   — Factors Influencing Insulin Secretion
      Substrates
      Hormonal Influences on Insulin Secretion
      Gastrointestinal Tract and Insulin Secretion
      Central Nervous System
      Concluding Statement about Insulin Secretion and Its
      Control, Revised 1969
   — Transport of Insulin in Blood
   — Inactivation and Excretion of Insulin

   b. *Distribution of Insulin-Like Activity in Serum Proteins*
   c. *Interaction of Serum Proteins and Crystalline Insulin Preparations*
   d. *Serum Insulin Antagonists*
       Synalbumin Insulin Antagonist on Muscle Tissue
       Insulin Antagonists on Adipose Tissue
       Insulin Antagonists on Diabetic Acidosis
   e. *Insulin Biosynthesis*
   f. *Insulin Synthesis*
   g. *Insulin Structure and Activity Relationships*
   h. *Insulin Degradation*
   i. *Nature of Circulating Serum Insulin*
   j. *Comparison of Serum Insulin-Like Activity and Serum Immuno-reactive Insulin*
   k. *Serum Insulin-Like Activity in Diabetes*
       Diaphragm and Adipose Tissue Assays
       Serum 'Bound Insulin' in Diabetes
       Atypical or Nonsuppressible Insulin in Diabetes
       Insulin Augmentation Effect in Diabetes
   l. *Pancreatic Insulin*
   m. *Serum Insulin Response to Insulin Stimulators in Diabetes*
       Sulfonylureas
       Biguanides
       Protein
       Hormones
       Other Material Influencing Insulin Secretion
   n. *Serum Insulin in Fetus and Neonate*
       Pregnancy and Serum Insulin Responses
   o. *Insulin in Urine*
   p. *Insulin Resistance*
       Classification
       Diagnosis
       Treatment
       Natural Course

5. GLUCAGON
   a. *Historical Background*
   b. *Chemcial Properties*
   c. *Source and Fate of Glucagon*
   d. *Role of Glucagon in Metabolism*
       Carbohydrate Metabolism
       Protein Metabolism
       Lipid Metabolism

e. *Effects of Glucagon*
        In Diabetes
        Effects on Cardiac Function
        Effects on Mineral Metabolism and Renal Function
        Effect on Gastrointestinal Tract
        Effect on Skin
        Role in Pancreatitis (Acute Hemorrhagic)
f. *Neoplasms Containing Glucagon*
g. *Glucagon Deficiency*
h. *Current Clinical Uses of Glucagon*
i. *Summary*

6. GLYCOPROTEINS AND DIABETIC MICROANGIOPATHY
    a. *Distribution and Structural Characteristics of Glycoproteins*
            Distribution
            Structure
    b. *Chemistry of the Glomerular Basement Membrane*
            Chemical Composition
            Structure
    c. *Chemistry of the Lesions of Diabetic Glomerulosclerosis*
            Histochemistry
            Chemical Analysis
    d. *Metabolism of Glycoproteins*
    e. *Metabolism of Glycoproteins in Diabetes*
    f. *Clinical Considerations*

7. THE PATHOLOGY OF DIABETES
    a. *Pancreas*
        —   The Normal Pancreas
        —   Microscopic Changes in the Islets of Langerhans
        —   Gross Pancreatic Changes
    b. *Kidney*
    c. *The Eye*
    d. *The Nervous System*
    e. *Cardiovascular Disease*
    f. *Endocrine Glands*
    g. *Miscellaneous Tissues and Organs*
    h. *Hemochromatosis*
    i. *Infants of Diabetic Mothers*
    j. *Diabetes and Infection*
    k. *Cancer and Diabetes*

l. *Pathological Effects of Oral Hypoclycemic Agents*
m. *Hyperinsulinism and Hypoglycemia*
n. *Autopsy Diagnosis of Diabetes and Hypoglycemia*
o. *Causes of Death*

8. LABORATORY PROCEDURES USEFUL IN DIAGNOSIS AND TREATMENT
   a. *Examination of the Urine*
      Volume of Urine in a 24-Hour Period
      Specific Gravity
      — Examination for Sugar
         Sugars of Normal Urine
         Sugar in Urine of a Diabetic Patient
         Qualitative Tests for Sugar
         Quantitative Tests
         Substances in Urine Causing Confusion in Testing for Sugar
      — Methods for the Determination of 'Ketone Bodies' in the Urine
         Qualitative Tests
         Quantitative Tests
      — Other Urine Tests
         Reaction of Urine
         Ammonia
         Nitrogen
         Albumin
         Casts
   b. *Examination of the Blood*
         Collection of Blood
         Automated Procedures
      — Blood Glucose
         Use of Plasma Versus Whole Blood
         Rapid Estimation of Blood Glucose
      — Carbon Dioxide in Blood Plasma
      — The Hydrogen-Ion Concentration of the Blood
      — Acetone in the Blood
         Method for Detection of Acetoacetic Acid and Acetone in the Blood
      — Other Blood Studies
   c. *Tests of Carbohydrate Tolerance*
         The Blood Glucose in Diabetic and Healthy Persons

- Current Mortality Statistics for the United States
  Age-Specific Death Rates by Color and Sex
  Mortality for Separate Racial Groups among the Colored
  Population, 1959-1961
  Regional Variations
  Comparison of Diabetes Mortality in Metropolitan and
  Nonmetropolitan Counties, 1959-1961
  Major Metropolitan Areas
  Mortality According to Marital Status
  Seasonal Variation in Mortality from Diabetes Mellitus
- Recent Mortality from Diabetes in Foreign Countries
- Trend in Diabetes Mellitus in the United States
  Trend of Age-Adjusted Rates, All Ages Combined, 1950-
  1967
  Trends by Age and Sex, 1950-1967
  Trends, 1920-1948
- Trends in Mortality from Diabetes in Foreign Countries since
  1950
- Socioeconomic Status and Occupation
  Mortality by Occupation—United States, 1950
  English Studies of Occupational Mortality

10. GENERAL PLAN OF TREATMENT AND DIET REGULATION
    a. *General Considerations*
    b. *Importance of Instruction of Patients, Their Families, and the Public*
    c. *Hospital Teaching Unit*
    d. *Dietary Standards*
    e. *Carbohydrate in the Body, Its Function and Uses*
    f. *Diabetic Diets*
       - Principles of Dietary Management
       - The Dietary Prescription
       - Standard Diets
       - Measurement of Food Values
         Estimation of Foods
         Measurement of Foods
         Weighing of Foods
         The Exchange System of Meal Planning
         Approximate Food Equivalents
         Sick-Day Diet
         Substitutions for School or Picnic Lunches

d. *Atypical Diabetes*
    Lipoatrophy
e. *Stages of the Diabetic State*
    Prediabetes
    Chemical Diabetes
f. *Nondiabetic Meliturias*
g. *Emotional and Behavior Problems*
h. *Prognosis*
i. *Histopathology*
j. *Diabetes Mellitus in Infants*
    Selection of Cases and Objectives
    Findings
    Treatment
    Diet
    Discharge from Hospital and Instructions to Parents

14. DIABETIC KETOACIDOSIS AND COMA
    a. *Incidence and Results of Treatment*
    b. *Clinical Features*
        Age and Sex
        Duration of Diabetes Prior to Coma
        Recurrent Episodes of Coma
        Hepatomegaly
    c. *Etiology*
        Exercise and Ketogenesis
    d. *Pathogenesis*
        Metabolic Changes in Uncontrolled Diabetes
        Ketogenesis
        Metabolic Effects of 'Ketoacids'
    e. *Hyperlipemia Associated with Grossly Uncontrolled Diabetes*
    f. *Effects of Uncontrolled Diabetes Upon Water and Electrolytes*
    g. *Metabolic Acidosis*
    h. *Prevention or Delay in Development of Decompensated Ketoacidosis*
        Water Balance
        Prevention of Acidemia (Lowered pH)
        Compensatory Mechanisms
    i. *Decompensated Ketoacidosis and Coma*
        Symptoms and Signs
    j. *Laboratory Findings in Diabetic Coma*
        Blood
        Electrocardiogram

c. *Retinitis Proliferans*
    — Treatment of Retinitis Proliferans
        Pituitary Ablation
        Photocoagulation of the Retina
    — Intraocular Pressure and Retinitis Proliferans
d. *Other Ocular States*
        Transitory Refractive Changes
        Pupils
        Ophthalmoplegia
        Cataract
        Glaucoma
        Asteroid Hyalitis
        Lipemia Retinalis

17. DIABETIC NEPHROPATHY
    a. *Pyelonephritis and Urinary Tract Infection*
        Acute Pyelonephritis
        Chronic Pyelonephritis
        Asymptomatic Bacteriuria
        Pyelonephritis in Diabetes
        Treatment in Acute and Chronic Pyelonephritis
        Emphysematous Pyelonephritis (Pneumonephrosis, Renal
            Pneumatosis)
        Perinephric Abscess
        Cystitis
        Neuropathic Bladder
        Cystic Emphysematosa and Pneumaturia
    b. *Renal Medullary Necrosis*
    c: *Renal Cortical Necrosis*
    d. *Clinical Picture of Diabetic Nephropathy*
    e. *Diagnosis of Diabetic Nephropathy*
    f. *Clinical Factors in the Development of Diabetic Nephropathy*
    g. *Uremia and Insulin Requirements*
    h. *Carbohydrate Intolerance in Uremic Patients ('Azotemic Pseudo-
        diabetes')*
    i. *Clinicopathologic Correlation of Diabetic Neuropathy*
    j. *Course and Prognosis of Diabetic Nephropathy*
    k. *Prevalence of Diabetic Nephropathy*
    l. *Therapy of Diabetic Nephropathy*
        Kidney Transplants

m. *The Pathogenesis of Diabetic Microangiography and Diabetic Nephropathy*
    Angiopathy in Secondary Diabetes
    Diabetic Angiopathy in Experimental Animals
    Immunologic Mechanisms

18. THE NERVOUS SYSTEM AND DIABETES
    a. *Peripheral Nervous System*
        Pathology
        Chemistry
        Clinical Observations
    b. *Autonomous Nervous System*
        Visceral Neuropathy
    c. *Diabetic Amyotrophy*
    d. *Spinal Syndromes*
    e. *Insulin and Hypoglycemia*
    f. *Ketoacidosis*
    g. *Central Nervous System*
    h. *Congenital and Infectious Diseases*
        Congenital Anomalies
        Mucormycosis
    i. *Cerebrospinal Fluid*
    j. *Treatment of Neurologic Disorders*
        Cerebrovascular Syndromes
        Diabetic Neuropathy

19. PREGNANCY AND DIABETES
    Prevalence
    Material
    Diabetogenic Effect of Pregnancy
    Diagnosis
    Effect of Pregnancy upon the Course of Diabetes
    Effect of Pregnancy upon the Complications of Diabetes
    Effect of Diabetes upon the Course of Pregnancy
    Effect of Diabetes upon the Infant
    Management Programs
    Follow-up of the Child of a Diabetic
    Malignant Angiopathy and Pregnancy
    Conclusion

m. *Treatment of Other Lower Extremity Problems*
  Calluses, Corns, Warts, and Fungal Infections
  Night Cramps
  Buerger's Exercises
n. *Prevention of Infections and Gangrene*
  — Instructions for Care of the Feet Given to Diabetic Adults at the Joslin Clinic and the New England Deaconess Hospital
o. *Burns*

21. INFECTIONS AND DIABETES
  a. *Exacerbating Effect of Diabetes on the Course of Infection*
    Effect of Sugar Content
    Effect of Dehydration
    Effect of Malnutrition
    Humoral Factors
    Cellular Response
    Influence of Endocrine Systems
    Vascular Insufficiency
    Neuropathy
  b. *Infection in the Pathogenesis of Diabetes*
    Pancreatitis
  c. *Specific Infections and Localization of Infection in Diabetes*
    Osteomyelitis
    Tuberculosis
    Fungal Infections
    Nonclostridial Gas Infections
  d. *The Management of Infection in Diabetes*

22. DISORDERS OF THE BLOOD
  a. *The Anemias*
    — Anemias with Diabetes-Related Causes
      Diabetic Nephropathy
      Gastrointestinal Neuropathy with Malabsorption
      Anemia after Hypophysectomy
      Hemochromatosis
    — Anemias not Directly Related to Diabetic Causes
      Pernicious Anemia
      The Hymoloytic Anemias
      Iron Deficiency Anemia
  b. *Blood Groups*
  c. *Coagulation Defects in Diabetes*

Language in Society

PUBLISHED BY CAMBRIDGE UNIVERSITY PRESS

Editor Professor Dell Hymes
Graduate School of Education/C1
University of Pennsylvania
Philadelphia, PA 19104
Telephone: (215) 898-7369

Dr. Charles Rosenberg
Center for Advanced Study *in the* & Behavioral
Sciences
202 Junipero Serra Boulevard
Stanford, CA 94305

June 7, 1984

RE: Kahn, <u>Modes of medical instruction.</u>

Dear Dr. Rosenberg,

Thank you for agreeing to write a few paragraphs (on the above book. *(max. 300 words)* It is enclosed along with a copy of our style sheet and two copyright forms. Please complete the latter and return one with your notice. The other is for your files.

Sincerely yours,

Cherie Francis

Cherie Francis
Editorial Assistant

           Insulin Resistance in Acromegalics with Diabetes
           Hypopituitarism
    — The Thyroid Gland and Diabetes
           Theories and Experimental Studies in 'Thyrodiabetes'
    — Hyperthyroidism
           Incidence of Diabetes in Hyperthyroid Patients
           Diabetes Complicated by Hypothyroidism
           Incidence of Hyperthyroidism in Diabetes
           Priority in Appearance of Diabetes and Hyperthyroidism
           The Diagnosis of Diabetes in Hyperthyroidism
           Age of Diabetics with Hyperthyroidism
           Sex Incidence in Diabetics with Hyperthyroidism
           Diagnosis of Hyperthyroidism
           Laboratory Tests
           Treatment
    — Hypothyroidism
    — Miscellaneous Thyroid Disorders
  b. *The Adrenals and Diabetes*
    — Adrenal Cortex
           Adrenocortical Hypofunction (Addison's Disease)
           Adrenocortical Hyperfunction
    — Adrenal Medulla
  c. *Diabetes Insipidus and Diabetes Mellitus*
  d. *The Parathyroid Gland and Diabetes*
  e. *The Gonads and Diabetes*

25. CANCER AND DIABETES
  a. *Incidence of Cancer in Diabetic Patients*
  b. *Incidence of Diabetes Among Persons with Cancer*
  c. *Cases of Cancer and Diabetes in Joslin Clinic Series*
  d. *Cancer of the Pancreas*
        Incidence
        Diagnosis
        Relationship between Cancer of the Pancreas and Diabetes

26. ALLERGY AND DIABETES
  a. *Allergy to Insulin*
  b. *Treatment of Insulin Hypersensitivity*
  c. *Allergic Diseases in Diabetics*

Population Studies
Obesity and Other Factors
Effect of Varying Blood Sugar on Uric Acid Excretion
Pathogenesis of Gout
Treatment

c. *Diseases of the Musculoskeletal System and Diabetes*
Diabetic Osteopathy
Bursitis and Periarthritis
Osteoarthritis
Dupuytren's Contracture
Sudeck's Atrophy
Hyperostotic Spondylosis

d. *Lower Urinary Tract and Genital Disorders in Diabetes*
Urinary Tract Calculi
Disorders of the Prostate Gland
Cystic Emphysematosa
Calcification of the Vas Deferens

e. *Trace Metals, Cations, and Diabetes*
Magnesium
Chromium
Manganese
Cobalt
Potassium
Calcium
Iron
Copper
Molybdenum
Other Trace Metals

f. *Transplantation of the Pancreas*

29. EMOTIONAL FACTORS IN DIABETES MELLITUS

a. *Review of the Literature*
Direct Effects of Emotions upon Carbohydrate Metabolism
Indirect Effects of Emotions upon Diabetes
Meaning of Diabetes to the Individual Patient

b. *Emotional Factors in Diabetes in Adults*
Personality Types and Diabetes Mellitus
Clinical Examples
Pregnancy
Complications of Diabetes

Pathology
Pathogenesis
Clinical Picture and Diagnosis
Treatment
d. *Liver Disease and Hypoglycemia*
Pathogenesis
Clinical Picture
Treatment
e. *Galactosemia and Glycogen Storage Diseases*
f. *Ethanol-Induced Hypoglycemia*
Pathogenesis
Clinical Picture
Diagnosis
Treatment
g. *Endocrinopathies Associated with Hypoglycemia*
Anterior Pituitary Gland
Adrenal Cortex
Thyroid Gland
Pancreatic Alpha Cells
h. *Reactive Hypoglycemia*
Reactive Functional Hypoglycemia
Reactive Hypoglycemia Secondary to Early Diabetes
Dumping Syndrome
Leucine Sensitivity
Hereditary Fructose Intolerance
i. *Exogenous Hypoglycemia*
Iatrogenic Hypoglycemia
Factitious Hypoglycemia

32. NONDIABETIC MELITURIA
a. *Classification*
b. *Diabetes Mellitus and Potential Diabetes*
Diabetes Mellitus
Potential Diabetes
c. *Nondiabetic Glycosuria*
Renal Glycosuria
Glycosuria of Pregnancy
Unclassified Glycosuria
Prognosis in Nondiabetic Glycosuria
d. *Melituria Other Than Glycosuria*
Chronic Essential Pentosuria

Fructosuria (Levulosuria)
Essential Fructosuria
Hereditary Fructose Intolerance
Familial Fructose and Galactose Intolerance
Lactosuria
Galactosuria
Mannoheptulosuria
Other Meliturias

b.   'POPULAR' TYPE: *DIABETES WITHOUT FEAR*[1]

The following 'key headings' include all nine chapter headings (see Arabic numerals) and their various subheadings[2] (indicated by alphabetical letters).

1. *Fiction Versus Fact*
    a. The misunderstood disease
    b. Scare stories
    c. Diabetic neurosis
    d. The fear worse than the disease
    e. Case histories
    f. Sources of misinformation
    g. Real-life success stories
    h. Putting the fears to rest
    i. The rational approach

2. *Basic Questions and Answers*
    a. Education and the diabetic
    b. Who should educate?
    c. The role of the doctor
    d. What is diabetes?
    e. What is insulin?
    f. The insulin numbering system
    g. Refrigerating insulin
    h. Air bubbles
    i. Rotating injection sites
    j. Best insulin dosage
    k. Changing the dosage
    l. Number of injections
    m. Insulin reaction
    n. Coping with hypoglycemia
    o. Oral drugs

3. *Keeping Control*
   a. Uselessness of complex self-testing methods
   b. Needless worry
   c. What is 'normal' blood sugar?
   d. The natural fluctuation of blood sugar levels
   e. 'Permissable' glucose levels
   f. The importance of testing
   g. Confusions from blood and urine self-testing
   h. Drawbacks of hospital tests
   i. The recommended procedure
   j. Freedom from worry

4. *Food and Drink*
   a. Nutritional neurosis and food faddism
   b. So-called 'forbidden' foods
   c. Guilt and anxiety
   d. Unnatural strictures on food and drink
   e. The medical evidence: sweets and alcohol are not in themselves harmful to diabetics
   f. Nature and history of diabetes
   g. Cumulative misinformation
   h. Sugar in the mouth does not mean sugar in the blood
   i. Medical studies
   j. The drawbacks of 'diabetic diets'
   k. Proliferation of hard-to-follow diets
   l. The best approach
   m. If the patient is underweight
   n. If the patient is overweight
   o. Normal weight
   p. Additional meals
   q. 'Diabetic foods'
   r. Alcohol
   s. The Goodman 'Meat Unlimited' Diet

5. *Marriage and Children*
   a. Emotional problems of diabetes
   b. Over-protective families
   c. Case histories
   d. The myth of hereditary diabetes
   e. The myth of dangerous pregnancies
   f. Where the myths came from

g. History of diabetes treatment
h. The truth about safe pregnancy
i. The truth about heredity

6. *Complications*
   a. Misinformation about medical complications
   b. The negative approach
   c. Half-truths and exaggerations
   d. The hospital and diabetes
   e. The positive aspects of diabetes
   f. The truth about infection
   g. Wound healing
   h. Atherosclerosis
   i. Diabetic neuropathy
   j. Eyesight
   k. Dental complications
   l. Kidney damage
   m. Foot lesions
   n. Other medical complications
   o. Needless fears
   p. The healthy diabetic

7. *Diabetes in Children*
   a. Emotional stress
   b. Problems of the adolescent
   c. Fearful parents
   d. Overcoming family guilt
   e. Overcoming popular misinformation
   f. Insulin and children
   g. The child's responsibility
   h. Diet and exercise
   i. Honesty and the child
   j. Emotional growth
   k. The role of the teacher
   l. Health attitudes
   m. Overprotection

8. *Research*
   a. The Juvenile Diabetes Association
   b. The American Diabetes Association
   c. Research in prevention

    d. New diagnostic techniques
    e. Improving insulin effectiveness
    f. Insulin delivery
    g. Monitoring the system
    h. Artificial pancreas
    i. Pancreas transplants
    j. Transplantation of cells
    k. The research jigsaw puzzle

9. *The Positive Approach*
    a. Knowledge and self-assurance
    b. Turning a negative into a positive
    c. Personal testimonials

NOTES

1. Dr. Joseph I. Goodman, *Diabetes Without Fear* (New York: Avon, 1979).
2. The numerous bold-type headings dispersed throughout the chapters have not been included here as they roughly correspond to the subheadings included with the Table of Contents.

Communications from Textbook Editors

In December 1978, a separate letter was sent out to the editors of each of the three selected textbooks—T-1, T-2 and T-3—in which the writer posed the following questions:

1. In which journals are book reviews of your textbook to be found?
2. Can you send me information concerning the history of your textbook?
3. What factors determine the amount of space which is allotted to each topic in a textbook?

The editors of T-1 and T-2 (but not T-3) responded, and their letters (with enclosures) are reproduced on the following pages.

ENCLOSURE

THE BIRTH AND INFANCY OF A TEXTBOOK (TRH)[1]

The first edition (1950)

In the late summer of 1945, Morris Fishbein telephoned Tinsley Harrison (TH). Morris explained that he, himself, having recently retired as Editor of the JAMA,[2] had become scientific consultant to Doubleday which had just recently purchased the Blakiston Company of Philadelphia. The new owners wished to produce a book on Internal Medicine in order to compete with Cecil, published by Saunders. Cecil had come to enjoy an almost complete monopoly in the United States. It was suggested that TH come to New York and discuss with Fishbein and with Ted Phillips, the chief executive of Blakiston, the question of becoming editor-in-chief of the projected book. All expenses would be paid, there would be a small honorarium and tickets to the two most popular shows on Broadway would be provided.

TH stated that he thought that Cecil was out-of-date and that there was no textbook which presented the subject of internal medicine in a manner comparable to the way it was actually taught in the better medical schools. He had certain definite ideas concerning a different arrangement and a more modern approach to the subject. However he had neither the desire nor the time to edit such a book.

Fishbein stated that the trip to New York would involve no obligation whatever other than an open mind and willingness to transmit his ideas about a new arrangement as well as his thoughts concerning possible editors. After such discussions TH would be entirely free to decline if he so wished. Since these conditions seemed reasonable the invitation was accepted. TH would arrive in the late afternoon, attend the theater and join Morris Fishbein and Ted Phillips for breakfast and lunch. After an afternoon matinee he would take an early evening flight back to Dallas where he was then chairman of the Department of Medicine at the Southwestern Medical College.

Upon being introduced to Ted Phillips at breakfast, TH was most favorably impressed. Here was personal charm, a rapid grasp of new ideas and a quick insight not only into features of a book that might facilitate its sales but also that might enhance its intellectual value to the reader.

The discussions were initially centered on arrangement. All agreed that the arrangement of current textbooks was outmoded. They had changed little since the first edition of Osler had appeared one-half century earlier. At that time nothing was known about the physiology and biochemistry of disease.

GEORGE W. THORN, M.D.
45 Shattuck Street
Boston, Massachusetts 02115
Tel.: 617-734-3300

Hersey Professor of the
Theory and Practice of Physic,
Emeritus
Harvard Medical School

Physician-in-Chief,
Emeritus
Peter Bent Brigham Hospital

January 4, 1979

Joan Kahn
McGill University
Graduate Program in Communications
815 Sherbrooke Street West
Montreal, PQ, Canada H3A2K6

Dear Ms. Kahn:

In regard to your first question, I would suggest that you
write to Mr. Dereck Jeffers at McGraw-Hill Book Company,
1221 Avenue of the Americas, New York 10020, who could provide you directly with the medical journals which have
book reviewed the 8th edition of the book.

I am enclosing a brief account of the early founding of
the Textbook and would state that there was a group of
six editors who share equal responsibility of the development of six sections of the Textbook.

In answer to your third question, it was felt that those
areas which move more rapidly in terms of medical advance
deserve more space and those areas which are more or
less stationary are reduced, in order to keep the book
a compassable size. Highly specialized areas, such as
eye, skin, etc. are largely taken care of by references
except for those disturbances which are of immediate importance to the internist or general practitioner.

I trust these comments will be of assistance.

Sincerely yours,

George W. Thorn, M.D.

rlk
enc.

Hence clinical medicine was mainly empirical and related to morbid anatomy and, in lesser degree, to mircrobiology. Much was known concerning the 'what' of disease and diagnosis but almost nothing about the 'why' and about treatment.

During the ensuing fifty years a revolution had occurred. A major faction of our teaching was now devoted to pathophysiology and pathochemistry. Since these topics related to reversible alterations in function rather than irreversible changes in structure, a knowledge of them was a fundamental first step in treatment if it was to be based on reason rather than on rote. But against such heresies the textbooks of medicine had remained as firm as Gibraltar, unshaken by the winds of change, and uneroded by the rains of progress.

Patients do not usually come to physicians with known diseases. Rather, they come with complaints or symptoms. Likewise many of them present abnormal physical signs. It is these manifestations of disease, the signs, and especially the symptoms, that provide the initial clues to the underlying disease; i.e. the clues to diagnosis. Therefore a textbook should begin with a consideration of the major manifestations of internal disorders and, after that, proceed to discussion of specific diseases.

Both of the hosts expressed strong agreement with these ideas concerning arrangement. This was not surprising. Feeling that he had thus repaid his obligation and sung for his supper, TH proceeded to discussion of what he deemed to be the entirely unacceptable conditions that would be necessary for him to consider the editorship.

There would need to be an editorial board which TH would select. This group would personally write much, perhaps most, of the book. They would have a free hand in selecting such additional authors as they deemed necessary. In choosing editors and authors there should be no consideration except the intellectual quality of the book. Thus the tendency, then current to some textbooks and systems of medicine, to pay large attention to a wide geographic distribution with one or more writers from practically every medical school, in order to augment sales, would not be followed.

Then came the surprising statement. Ted Phillips said, and Fishbein agreed, that they concurred completely with the idea of disregarding geographic distribution and other considerations of medical politics in choosing authors. They were heartily in favor of one criterion only — the probable contribution of an individual to the quality of the book.

TH now felt that he had been partially disarmed. He had counted heavily on his assumption that the publisher would insist on including members of the faculty of most of the medical schools as a means of assuring large sales.

He had thought that there would develop an irreconcilable difference on this point and that this disagreement would justify his polite withdrawal from the venture. Although his disinclination to participate was being weakened by the completely cooperative attitude of Fishbein and Phillips and by what seemed to be a fine insight into what the projected book should be, TH was not, as yet, convinced that he wished to undertake the job. He still had in his arsenal certain weapons that might induce the publisher to prefer a different editor-in-chief.

There would need to be fairly frequent, brief meetings of the editors with the publisher and with each other. In addition, it was desirable that there be occasional longer meetings lasting for perhaps ten days to two weeks.

TH stated that while he was still reluctant to become editor-in-chief it might be fruitful to consider possible individuals to be selected as editors. He added that in his opinion at least one of them should be a person actively engaged in the private practice of medicine. If the proper type of person could be obtained he would tend to introduce a feet-on-the-ground point of view and keep the other editors, presumably academicians, from producing a volume too far removed from the realities of day-by-day patient care.

VETERANS ADMINISTRATION
Hospital
4435 BEACON AVENUE SO.
SEATTLE, WASHINGTON   98108

January 3, 1978

IN REPLY
REFER TO:

Ms. Joan Kahn
Graduate Program in Communications
McGill University
Macdonald-Harrington Building
Montreal, PQ
Canada   H3A 2K6

Dear Ms. Kahn:

I have your inquiry about the Textbook of Medicine edited by Dr. McDermott and myself, and I will try to help you some with the information you want.

As to book reviews of the Textbook, I don't have any, nor could I give you a partial list of places in which they have appeared. I think, however, that you might have better luck writing to the publishers and I suggest you write to Mr. John J. Hanley, W.B. Saunders Company, West Washington Square, Philadelphia, Pennsylvania 19105, and say that I referred you to him. The fact is, though, the book reviews of a new edition of an established textbook that has been in use for a half a century, are not very educational reading. The book is huge, over two thousand pages, and the usual type of review simply says another edition has appeared, that it weighs so many pounds, etc. It may also paraphrase some of the remarks in the Preface in which the editors make some general remarks about changes that have been made since the preceding edition.

There is no "history" of this Textbook that I know of. I have been toying with the idea of trying to write one, using it as a framework to illustrate how new clinical knowledge is derived. You will find a little bit of history in the Preface to the current (14th) Edition. I am also enclosing a semi-final draft of the Preface we have prepared for the 15th Edition which will be published in March. The wording has been changed a little bit, but this will be unimportant for your purposes.

Your third question is a difficult one, i.e., the factors that might influence the amount of space allotted to each subspecialty. We look on this Textbook as a sort of lexicon to which a medical student or practicing physician can turn for at least some information on almost any disease or syndrome that he hears mentioned. For the rarer entities, we devote comparatively little space, but try to add references at the end of each chapter that will give the interested person an entry point into the literature so that he can obtain fuller information from primary sources. Obviously, we cannot be guided entirely by the frequency or

"To care for him who shall have borne the battle, and for his widow, and his orphan." – ABRAHAM LINCOLN

gravity of a given illness. If frequency were the determining factor,
then about two-thirds of the book would be given over to common
respiratory infections and to acute gastrointestinal upsets. The
decision about space allocation is perhaps the most important function
of the editors, who must take an overall view of the book, and who
must find some way to cram some information about everything between
two hard covers. We have nine associate editors and have meetings
with them in which we go over new subjects to be included in each
edition and the relative number of pages that can be allocated to
each subspecialty. In our letters of invitation to contributors, we
are very specific about the number of words, translated into text pages,
and as a general rule they are quite faithful about adhering to the
guidelines.

The most difficult problem of the editors is to get things in on
time. We give each contributor a very definite deadline date for
receipt of the manuscript and we nearly always send him or her a
reminder letter about two months in advance of that deadline. We
set the deadlines more or less in order of appearance in the Textbook,
as the printers like to work forward from the beginning to the end
of the book. When dealing with 200 contributors gathered about the
world, we are bound to run into some delinquents and in such cases we
employ a variety of tactics including telephone calls and telegrams
and, if necessary, we sometimes have to persuade a local colleague
to write the chapter quickly and forget about someone who is having
so much difficulty with a psychological depression or a divorce or
myocardial infarction, that he just can't write his promised chapter.

I hope this will be some help to you and I hope, also, I will have an
opportunity to see your thesis when it is completed.

Sincerely yours,

Paul B. Beeson

Encl.

-2-

ENCLOSURE

PREFACE

What is a textbook? It is a putting-together of discrete pieces of information into a cohesive, meaningful pattern. In the weaving of this pattern, the editors of this Fifteenth Edition of the *Textbook of Medicine* have been mindful as in the previous editions of the original purposes of Russell Cecil and Robert Loeb to provide authoritative clinical guidance and a reasoned, scientific basis for the pursuit of medicine. The two ideas are complementary, for an understanding of the mechanisms of disease and its manifestations enables the physician to select appropriate diagnostic procedures and therapy. This guiding principle is underscored by introducing each major section with an overview of pathophysiology and the principles of approach to the clinical problem.

The period of time covered by editions of this textbook extends from 1927, soon after the epochal discoveries of insulin for diabetes and the liver treatment of pernicious anemia, through an era of unprecedented effort in biomedical research and clinical investigation; hence each succeeding edition has required substantial revision to keep pace with emerging knowledge and technology. The first edition came to about 800,000 words and had 130 contributors. The present edition runs well over 2,000,000 words and has more than 200 contributors. The number of individual clinical entities and syndromes has grown from about 550 in the first edition to an almost unaccountable number in the current edition. For example, the subject of intestinal malabsorption, of which 41 forms are now described, was dealt with only under the term 'tropical sprue' in 1927. Sickle cell anemia was given a nine-line paragraph in the first edition; there are now five chapters dealing with disorders associated with 180 different hemoglobins. The diagnostic procedures available in 1927 were relatively simple and crude (blood sugar, blood urea nitrogen, x-ray, and the use of rigid endoscopes). Modern diagnostic capabilities are, by comparison, immensely refined, including such precise aids as angiography, ultrasound, and computerized tomography, together with many new chemical determinations, some so delicate that they can measure hormone concentrations in picagram quantities.

Our therapeutic capabilities have similarly expanded. In 1927 two favorite drugs, arsenic (Fowler's solution) and potassium iodide, were each recommended for 30 to 40 different diseases. The current edition discusses the use of scores of effective and well-tested compounds, along with such high technologies as renal dialysis, parenteral nutrition, platelet transfusion, assisted respiration, and cardiac pacemakers. Surgery of the heart has revolutionized the practice of cardiology, and the replacement of joints has gained an established place in the field of rheumatology.

The flow of new ideas and new procedures continues, as reflected in this new edition. Several major Parts have been completely revised and rewritten: diseases of the respiratory tract, cardiovascular diseases, renal diseases, bone diseases, and skin diseases. Indeed, all continuing chapters have been revised to a greater or lesser extent to fit today's situation.

Several new Parts have been added. First is one on Human Growth and Development. The remarkable lengthening in average life-span that is taking place in this century calls for greater textbook emphasis on the changes that occur over time in the structure and function of the human body. Inasmuch as older patients make disproportionate demands on health services, it can be predicted that when our present medical students and house officers reach mid-career, about half their work will be in the care of people over the age of 65 years.

A new Part - Critical Care Medicine — has been made necessary by advances both in the understanding and in the technology of supportive measures for failing respiratory cardiac or renal function. Coronary Care Units and Medical Intensive Care Units are now commonplace in general hospitals and the specialty of Critical Care Medicine has emerged. Inevitably, some of the matters discussed in this Part must also be mentioned in other chapters; nevertheless, it seemed desirable to bring together a general discussion of the principles of this kind of treatment in a separate Part.

Oncology is now a formal subspecialty of internal medicine, with a rapidly expanding body of knowledge from research and from clinical experience. The editors felt it appropriate, therefore, to consolidate chapters on cancer into a new Part, to give the user easier access to information, and to underscore the importance of the subject in clinical practice.

Ocular manifestations accompany many systemic diseases and it was decided that this edition should include a Part dealing with those aspects of Ophthalmology that should be part of the working knowledge of the internist or primary care physician. Special emphasis is laid on the funduscopic changes that may provide clues to the existence or progress of such conditions as lupus erythematosus, leukemia, hypertension, and hereditary disorders.

Another new Part deals with the subject of Drug Interactions. Although the detail of this subject is immense, the editors believe that certain principles which underlie drug interactions, can be illustrated in examples and that they would be helpful to users of the book.

Diagnostic techniques have undergone remarkable changes since the last edition; consequently much more emphasis is given to the use of such procedures as fiberscopic endoscopy, ultrasound, computerized tomography, Doppler studies, nuclear imaging, and selective angiography.

This body of information is now so that the place of importance of each individual piece cannot be finally judged solely by the editors; they must have expert help. For Disorders of the Nervous System and Behavior there is a separate editor, Fred Plum. In addition, nine physicians widely recognized as expert authorities in particular branches of medicine have served as consulting editors: Alexander Bearn (Medical Genetics), Nicholas Christy (Diseases of the Endocrine System), Philip Marsden (Protozoan and Helminthic Diseases), John Murray (Respiratory Diseases), Ralph Nachman (Diseases of the Blood), Roscoe Robinson (Renal Diseases), Marvin Sleisenger (Diseases of the Digestive System), Andrew Wallace (Cardiovascular Diseases), and Sheldon Wolff (Microbial Diseases). A book is ideas made visible. This process could not have been accomplished without these consulting editors and the contributors. We are greatly indebted to them all for their selfless help.

In order to assist our users to cope with the increasing need for continuing medical education and recertification, a companion book and answers are being devised by members of the Departments of Medicine at Duke University and the University of California, San Francisco.

To have attempted to put the essence of contemporary medicine within the covers of this textbook, is an exciting and demanding adventure in which the three of us have joined as Co-Editors. For Beeson and McDermott this edition will be the last, and Wyngaarden will be joined by Lloyd H. Smith, Jr., as Co-Editor of the next edition. This change is in keeping with the book's history of orderly transition.

We cannot close without expressing our pleasure in the friendship and invaluable advice of Jack Hanley, Vice President and General Manager for Health Sciences of the W.B. Saunders Company. We wish also to thank the many other able and devoted people in the Company from whom we have learned so much. It is a special pleasure to acknowledge with gratitude the skill and untiring efforts of Dave Kilmer, Special Projects Editor at Sanders, who has so ably helped us to bring together this large assemblage of writings. Finally, we must acknowledge special indebtedness to Helen Miller, who has now been with the book for six editions, and to Patsey Sutphin, for whom this edition has been the first. Together these editorial assistants have done a splendid job not only in faultlessly handling hundreds of manuscripts and proofs, but in providing the linkage that binds contributors, publisher, consulting editors, and ourselves to the facts and ideals of medicine. Their help deserves, and has, our deepest thanks.

Paul B. Beeson
Walsh McDermott
James B. Wyngaarden

NOTES

1. Tinsley R. Harrison.
2. *Journal of the American Medical Association.*
3. Principles of *I*nternal Medicine.

Bibliography*

A. PRIMARY SOURCES

Beeson, Paul B. and Walsh McDermott. *Textbook of Medicine,* 14th ed. (Philadelphia: W.B. Saunders, 1975).
Cooley, D.G., ed. *Better Homes and Gardens Family Medical Guide,* Rev. ed. (New York: Meredith, 1977).
Fishbein, Morris, ed. *The Handy Home Medical Adviser and Concise Medical Encyclopedia,* New rev. ed. (New York: Doubleday, 1973).
Gerras, Charles et al., eds. *The Encyclopedia of Common Diseases.* (Emmaus, Penn.: Rodale, 1976).
Goodman, Joseph I. *Diabetes Without Fear.* (New York: Avon, 1979).
Harvey, Abner McGehee, ed. *The Principles and Practice of Medicine,* 19th ed. (New York: Appleton-Century-Crofts, 1976).
Homola, Samuel. *Doctor Homola's Natural Health Remedies.* (West Nyack, N.Y.: Parker, 1973).
Lehninger, Albert L. *Biochemistry,* 2nd ed. (New York: Worth, 1975).
Marble, Alexander et al., eds. *Joslin's Diabetes Mellitus.* (Philadelphia: Lea and Febiger, 1971).
Miller, Benjamin, and Laurence Galton. *The Family Book of Preventive Medicine: How to Stay Well All the Time.* (New York: Simon and Schuster, 1971).
Stedman's Medical Dictionary, 23rd ed. (Baltimore: Williams and Wilkins, 1976).
Thorn, George Widmer, ed. *Harrison's Principles of Internal Medicine,* 8th ed. (New York: McGraw Hill, 1977).
World Health Organization. *Manual of International Statistical Classification of Diseases, Injuries and Causes of Death.* Vol. 1. (Geneva: World Health Organization (United Nations), 1977).

B. SECONDARY SOURCES

Abrams, M.H. *A Glossary of Literary Terms,* 3rd ed. (New York: Holt, Rinehart and Winston, 1971).

Annan, Gertrude L. 'Medical Americana'. *Journal of the American Medical Association* 192 (12 April 1965): 139-144.

Annan, Gertrude L. and J.W. Felter, eds. *Handbook of Medical Library Practice*, 3rd ed. (Chicago: Medical Library Association, 1970).

Bellert, Irena. 'On various solutions of the problem of presuppositions', In *Studies in Text Grammar*, ed. by J.S. Petofi and H. Rieser, pp. 79-95. (Dordrecht, Holland: D. Reidel, 1973).

―― 'On references and interpretation of natural language sentences'. *Theoretical Linguistics* 1 (1974): 215-230.

Bellert, Irena, and Peter Ohlin, eds. *Selected Concepts in Semiotics and Aesthetics.* (Montreal: Programme in Communications, McGill University, 1978).

Black, Max. *Models and Metaphors: Studies in Language and Philosophy.* (Ithaca, N.Y.: Cornell University Press, 1962).

Blake, John B. 'From Buchan to Fishbein: The literature of domestic medicine'. In *Medicine Without Doctors*, ed. by Guenter B. Risse, Ronald L. Numbers, and Judith Wolzer Leavitt, pp. 11-29. (New York: Science History Publications, U.S.A., 1977).

Bogdonoff, Morton D. 'Book reviews'. *The New England Journal of Medicine* 301 (26 July 1979): 220.

Bunge, Mario. *Scientific Research 1: The Search for System.* (New York: Springer-Verlag, 1967).

Bussy, R. Kenneth, ed. *Philadelphia's Publishers and Printers: An Informal History.* (Philadelphia: Philadelphia Book Clinic, 1976).

Carson, Gerald. *One for a Man, Two for a Horse.* (Garden City, N.Y.: Doubleday, 1961).

Ching-Chih Chen. *Biomedical, Scientific and Technical Book Publishing.* (Metuchen, N.J.: Scarecrow, 1976).

Cronbach, Lee J. et al., eds. *Text Materials in Modern Education: A Comprehensive Theory and Platform for Research.* (Urbana, Ill.: University of Illinois Press, 1955).

Culler, Jonathan. *Saussure.* (Glasgow: William Collins, 1976).

Daniels, U. and S. White. *Medical Textbook Review* (Cambridge, England: Clinical School Offices, University of Cambridge, Adderbrooke's Hospital, 1976-).

Dirckx, John H. *The Language of Medicine: Its Evolution, Structure and Dynamics.* (Hagerstown, Ma.: Harper and Row, 1976).

Dubos, Rene. *Mirage of Health.* (New York: Doubleday, 1959).

Ducrot, Oswald, and Tzvetan Todorov. *Encyclopedic Dictionary of the Sciences of Language.* Trans. by Catherine Porter. (Baltimore: Johns Hopkins University Press, 1979).

Ebel, Robert E., ed. *Encyclopedia of Educational Research*, 4th ed. (London: Collier-Macmillan, 1969).

Edwards, Paul, ed. *The Encyclopedia of Philosophy.* Vol. 7. (New York: The Free Press, 1967).

Fleming, Thomas P., and Russell Shank. 'Scientific and technical book publishing . *Library Trends* 7 (July 1958): 197-209.

Harvey, Abner McGehee, and Victor A. McKusick, eds. *Osler's Textbook Revisited.* (New York: Appleton, 1967).

Hechtlinger, Adelaide. *The Great Patent Medicine Era or Without Benefit of Doctor.* (New York: Grosset and Dunlap, 1970).

Holsti, Ole R. *Content Analysis for the Social Sciences and Humanities.* (Reading, Mass.: Addison-Wesley, 1969).

Jacob, Francois. *The Logic of Life: A History of Heredity.* Trans. by Betty E. Spillman. (New York: Random House, 1976).

Johnson, Barbara Coe. 'Medical book publishing'. *Library Trends* 7 (July 1958): 210-219.

Joos, Martin. *The Five Clocks.* (Bloomington: Indiana University, Research Center in Anthropology, Folklore and Linguistics, 1962).

Keys, Thomas E. 'Some American medical imprints of the nineteenth century'. *Bulletin of the Medical Library Association* 45 (1957): 309-318.

King, Lester S. *The Growth of Medical Thought.* (Chicago: University of Chicago Press, 1963).

King, Lloyd W. and M. Frank Redding. 'Textbook publishing'. *Library Trends* 7 (July 1958): 50-56.

Kuhn, Thomas S. *The Structure of Scientific Revolutions,* 2nd ed. International Encyclopaedia of Unified Science, vol. 2, no. 2 (Chicago: University of Chicago Press, 1939).

Lanham, Richard A. *A Handlist of Rhetorical Terms: A Guide for Students of English Literature.* (Berkeley and Los Angeles: University of California Press, 1968).

Leech, Geoffrey. *Semantics.* (Middlesex: Penguin, 1974).

Lewis, Kathleen. 'Conference on language and medicine'. *Language Sciences* 12 (1970): 14-16.

Lieb, I.C., ed. *Charles S. Peirce's Letters to Lady Welby.* (New Haven: Whitlock's, 1953).

Locke, John. *An Essay Concerning Human Understanding.* Abr. and ed. by A.D. Woozley. (New York: Collins, 1964).

Lyons, John. *Introduction to Theoretical Linguistics.* (Cambridge, England: Cambridge University Press, 1968).

___ *Semantics:1.* (Cambridge, England: Cambridge University Press, 1977).

Magee, Bryan. *Karl Popper.* (New York: The Viking Press, 1973).

Mallery, Richard D. *Grammar, Rehetoric and Composition.* (New York: Doubleday, 1967).

Mates, Benson. *Stoic Logic.* (Berkeley: Universityof California Press, 1953).

McKeown, Thomas. *Medicine in Modern Society.* (New York: Hafner, 1966).

___ *The Role of Medicine: Dream, Mirage, or Nemesis?* (London: Nuffield Provincial Hospitals Trust, 1976).

Medical Books and Serials in Print 1979: An Index to Literature in the Health Sciences. (New York: Bowker, 1979).

Medical School Admission Requirements, 1979-1980. (Washington, D.C.: Association of American Colleges, 1978).

Miller, Jonathan. *The Body in Question.* (New York: Random House, 1978).

Morris, Charles. *Foundations of the Theory of Signs.* Vol. 1, no. 2 of *Foundations of the Unity of Science: Toward an International Encyclopedia of Unified Science.* (Chicago: University of Chicago Press, 1938).

Narin, Francis. *Evaluative Bibliometrics: The Use of Publication and Citation Analysis in the Evaluation of Scientific Activity.* (Cherry Hill, N.J.: Computer Horizons, 1976).

Notkins, Abner Louis. 'The causes of diabetes'. *Scientific American* 241 (November 1979): 62.

The Osler Library. (Montreal: McGill University, 1979).

Pollak, Kurt, in collaboration with E. Ashworth Underwood. *The Healers: The Doctor, Then and Now.* (London: Nelson, 1968).

Popper, Karl R. *Conjectures and Refutations: The Growth of Scientific Knowledge.* (New York: Harper and Row, 1965).

   Objective Knowledge: An Evolutionary Approach. (London: Oxford University Press, 1972).

   The Open Society and Its Enemies. Vol. 1. (London: Routledge and Kegan Paul, 1977).

Reichenbach, Hans. *Symbolic Logic.* (New York: Macmillan, 1947).

Reiser, S.J. *Medicine and the Reign of Technology.* (New York: Cambridge University Press, 1978).

Riese, Walther. *The Conception of Disease: Its History, Its Versions, and Its Nature.* (New York: Philosophical Library, 1953).

de Saussure, Ferdinand. *Course in General Linguistics.* (New York: McGraw-Hill, 1966).

Sebeok, Thomas, ed. *Studies in Semiotics: Contributions to the Doctrines of Signs.* (Bloomington: Indiana University Press, 1976).

   The Tell-tale Sign: A Survey of Semiotics. (Lisse, Netherlands: Peter de Ridder Press, 1975).

Shapiro, Martin. *Getting Doctored: Critical Reflections on Becoming a Physician.* (Kitchener, Ont.: Between the Lines, 1978).

The Shorter Oxford English Dictionary on Historical Principles, 3rd ed. 2 vols. (Oxford: Clarendon, 1977).

Sontag, Susan. *Illness as Metaphor.* (New York: Farrar, Strauss and Giroux, 1977).

Swanson, Don R. 'Information retrieval as a trial and error process'. *Library Quarterly* 47 (April 1977): 128-148.

Temkin, Owsei. 'Health and disease'. In *Dictionary of the History of Ideas,* vol. 2, pp. 395-407. Ed. by Philip P. Wiener. 4 vols. (New York: Scribner, 1973).

Thornton, John L. *Medical Books, Libraries and Collectors.* (London: Andre Deutsch, 1966).

Tukey, John W. *Exploring Data Analysis.* (Reading, Mass.: Addison-Wesley, 1977).

UNESCO. Classification Research Group. *The Need for a Faceted Classification as the Basis of all Methods of Information Retrieval.* Document 320/5515, 1955.

Wartman, William B. *Medical Teaching in Western Civilization: A History Prepared from the Writings of Ancient and Modern Authors.* (Chicago: Year Book Medical Publishers, 1961).

Who's Who in America 1976-1977. 39th ed. 2 vols. (Chicago: Marquis Who's Who, 1978).

Who's Who in America 1978-1979. 40th ed. Chicago: Marquis Who's Who, 1978.

Who's Who in Health Care, 1st ed. (New York: Hanover, 1977).

Wolfe, Gerard R. 'The Appletons: Four generations of publishing in America'. Ph.D. dissertation, Union Graduate School, 1978.

Index

Tasso Borbé (Editor)

Semiotics Unfolding

Proceedings of the Second Congress of the International
Association for Semiotic Studies, Vienna, July 1979

1984. 14,8 x 22,8 cm. 34 illustrations.
Volume I: XIV, 678 pages.
Volume II: XIV, pages 679–1268.
Volume III: XIV, pages 1269–1846.
Cloth, together DM 420,–; US $191.00
ISBN 3 11 009779 6 (Approaches to Semiotics 68)

The over 200 papers contained in these volumes were written
for the second international congress (IASS/AIS) to be officially
devoted to semiotics. They offer a representative overview of the
present state of theoretical development, empirical research, and
practical application of semiotics.

The contributions are naturally aimed at semioticians, but also
at everyone who wishes to become familiar with the semiotic concepts of experiencing, perceiving, understanding, describing, and
interpreting the world and its events.

Contents

Volume I

Part 1   Theory and History of Semiotics
Part 2   Semiotics and Social Interaction

Volume II

Part 3   Semiotics in Text and Literature
Part 4   Linguistics and Semiotics

Volume III

Part 5   Semiotics in Architecture and Fine Arts
Part 6   Semiotics and Visual Communication
Part 7   Semiotics in Theatre, Music, and Film

Prices are subject to change without notice

mouton publishers
Berlin · New York · Amsterdam